OXFORD MEDICAL PUBLICATIONS

Oxford Handbook of
Clinical
Rehabilitation

Second edition

Oxford Handbook of
Clinical
Rehabilitation

Second edition

Anthony B. Ward

Professor in Rehabilitation Medicine
University Hospital of North Staffordshire
North Staffordshire Rehabilitation Centre
Stoke on Trent, UK

Michael P. Barnes

Honorary Professor of Neurological Rehabilitation
Newcastle University;
Consultant Neurologist and Consultant in
Rehabilitation Medicine
Hunters Moor Neurorehabilitation Ltd,
Newcastle upon Tyne, UK

Sandra C. Stark

Consultant Therapist in Neurorehabilitation
Professional Lead
Walkergate Park International Centre for
Neurorehabilitation and Neuropsychiatry
Newcastle upon Tyne, UK

Sarah Ryan

Nurse Consultant Rheumatology
Staffordshire Rheumatology Centre
Stoke on Trent, UK

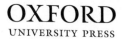

OXFORD
UNIVERSITY PRESS

OXFORD
UNIVERSITY PRESS

Great Clarendon Street, Oxford OX2 6DP

Oxford University Press is a department of the University of Oxford.
It furthers the University's objective of excellence in research, scholarship,
and education by publishing worldwide in

Oxford New York

Auckland Cape Town Dar es Salaam Hong Kong Karachi
Kuala Lumpur Madrid Melbourne Mexico City Nairobi
New Delhi Shanghai Taipei Toronto

With offices in

Argentina Austria Brazil Chile Czech Republic France Greece
Guatemala Hungary Italy Japan Poland Portugal Singapore
South Korea Switzerland Thailand Turkey Ukraine Vietnam

Oxford is a registered trade mark of Oxford University Press
in the UK and in certain other countries

Published in the United States
by Oxford University Press Inc., New York

© Oxford University Press, 2009

The moral rights of the authors have been asserted
Database right Oxford University Press (maker)

Previously published as Oxford Handbook of Rehabilitation Medicine 2005

Second edition published 2009

British Library Cataloguing in Publication Data
Data available

Library of Congress Cataloging-in-Publication-Data
Data available

Typeset by Cepha Imaging Private Ltd., Bangalore, India
Printed in China
on acid-free paper by
Asia Pacific Offset

ISBN 978-0-19-955052-4

10 9 8 7 6 5 4 3 2 1

Preface

We are delighted to include two new authors in this second edition—Sandra C. Stark and Sarah Ryan. We hope that this will make our handbook very applicable to a multidisciplinary readership which is, of course, essential to the proper delivery of rehabilitation. In the few years since we produced the first edition there continues to be expansion in rehabilitation. In recent years there have been further increases in the number of rehabilitation centres in the UK and indeed throughout Europe. We are also seeing the slow but gradual expansion of community-based rehabilitation teams that are so important for the ongoing rehabilitation of the disabled person once they leave the post-acute facility. We are also seeing diversification of rehabilitation with an increasing range of providers in the public, private, and not-for-profit sectors. This gives the disabled person more opportunity and more choice. However, there is no room for complacency and we are aware of the continuing patchy nature of rehabilitation provision in most countries.

We have updated this volume and produced a wider range of further reading lists. We hope that the book is still relevant for junior physicians as well as therapists, nurses, and clinical psychologists working in the field and we trust that it remains informative, useful and still imparts a sense of the real benefits that can accrue from a proper interdisciplinary rehabilitation programme.

Anthony B. Ward, Stoke on Trent
Michael P. Barnes, Newcastle upon Tyne
Sandra C. Stark, Newcastle upon Tyne
Sarah Ryan, Stoke on Trent
2009

Contents

Detailed contents

Concepts of rehabilitation

Introduction

What are the basic concepts of rehabilitation medicine? In many ways rehabilitation is different from most other medical specialties. It is primarily a process of education of the disabled person so that, ideally, they can cope with family, friends, work, and leisure with as little support as possible. Thus, rehabilitation is a process that centrally involves the disabled person in making plans and setting goals that are important and relevant to their own circumstances. Rehabilitation is not a process that is done *to* the disabled person but it is a process that is done *by* the disabled person with the guidance, support, and help of a wide range of professionals as well as family and friends. Rehabilitation is also a process that goes beyond the rather narrow confines of physical disease and also deals with the psychological consequences of disability as well as the social milieu in which the disabled person has to function. A key factor that differentiates rehabilitation from most of medicine is that it is not a process that can be carried out by medical practitioners alone and of necessity requires the active partnership of a whole range of health and social service professionals. The characteristics of rehabilitation are listed in Box 1.1.

Box 1.1 Characteristics of rehabilitation

- It is an educational process.
- Crucial involvement of the disabled person in programme planning.
- Key involvement of family, friends, and colleagues.
- It is a process that requires clear goals to be set and measured.
- It is a multidisciplinary process.
- It is a process based on the concepts of activity and participation—
  📖 see Impairment, activity, and participation p.4.

Impairment, activity, and participation

Historically, the key principles that lie behind rehabilitation are those that were proposed by the World Health Organization (WHO) in 1980—impairment, disability, and handicap. These old definitions are fundamental to rehabilitation and are shown in Box 1.2. However, whilst these older definitions are of significant historical interest, in 2001 they were replaced by new classifications produced by the WHO. The new definitions are seen in Box 1.3.

Impairment has remained in both these classifications. Impairment is simply a descriptive term that says nothing about consequence. A right hemiparesis, for example, or a left-sided sensory loss, or a homonymous hemianopia are impairments. However, the right hemiparesis can be relatively mild leading to virtually no functional consequence or can be profound leading to complete inability to walk. It is the functional consequence of the impairment that used to be described as the disability and is now described as activity limitation. Rehabilitation goes beyond impairment and looks at the functional context and tries to minimize the functional impact of such impairment. It is, after all, the limitation to activity that matters to the individual and not the impairment. Rehabilitation medicine does not minimize the importance of diagnosis and impairment in an effort to understand the underlying pathophysiology but simply places equal emphasis on the consequent limitation of activity.

Participation is defined as involvement in a life situation. This is broadly equivalent to the old term—handicap. Participation is described as social context. In our example of a right hemiparesis even a relatively mild right-sided weakness can have profound implications for a young man who is a scaffolder or who wanted to go into the armed services, as such occupations would be closed to him or an existing job may be lost. However, an older man who is already retired and whose abilities are restricted by other problems such a difficulty may have limited impact on his lifestyle. The concept of participation does not only deal with the broader physical consequence of an activity limitation but looks at the broader social context. A mild hemiparesis, for example, in a receptionist may not actually prevent that person from undertaking the job and being a good employee. However, the attitude of the employer to the disabled person may cause them to be moved elsewhere or even lose their job. A person who needs to use a wheelchair may be quite capable of undertaking their job but cannot move around the office because it is not wheelchair accessible. Rehabilitation needs to take into account not only the activity limitation but also the particular societal context for that person. Thus rehabilitation strays into the arena of societal attitudes and the physical environment, which are traditionally outside the realm of medicine.

Box 1.2 Historical definitions of the WHO's International Classification of Impairments, Disabilities and Handicaps (1980)

- *Impairment*: any loss or abnormality of psychological, physiological, or anatomical structure or function.
- *Disability*: any restriction or lack of activity resulting from an impairment to perform an activity in the manner or in the range considered normal for people of the same age, sex, and culture.
- *Handicap*: a disadvantage for a given individual resulting from impairment or disability that limits or prevents the fulfilment of a role that would otherwise be normal for that individual.

Box 1.3 International Classification of Functioning, Disability and Health (ICF)

- *Impairment*: loss or abnormality of a body structure or of a physiological or psychological function.
- *Activity*: the execution of a task or action by an individual. Thus, activity limitations are difficulties an individual may have in executing activities.
- *Participation*: involvement in a life situation and thus participation restrictions are problems an individual may experience in such involvement.
- *Environmental factors*: these make up the physical, social, and attitudinal environment in which people live and conduct their lives.
- *Contextual factors*: includes the features, aspects, and attributes of objects, structures, (participation) human-made organizations, service provision, and agencies in the physical, social, and attitudinal environment in which the people live and conduct their lives. Contextual factors include both environmental factors and personal factors.

Further details at www.who.int/classifications/icf

The full ICF is a complicated document, Basically, the scope of the ICF is to provide a description of situations with regard to human functioning. The ICF recognizes the importance not only of describing the functioning of an individual but also placing such functioning in to the social context. Fig 1.1 is taken from the WHO website and provides a useful summary.

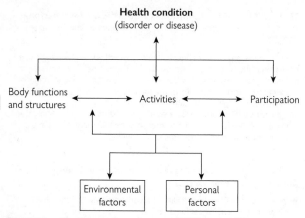

Fig 1.1 Interactions between the components of ICF. Reproduced from International Classification of Functioning, Disability and Health (ICF) ⍟ www.who. int/classifications/icf WHO press©, with permission.

Medical model of disability

The new classification of impairment, activity, and participation is a step towards a social model of disability and a step away from the medical model of disability. These terms are in common usage in the field of rehabilitation and need further description. The medical specialty of rehabilitation medicine has come from an 'illness' background. It has in the past been a specialism that in general has been carried out by physicians with the support of nurses and therapists and delivered to disabled people. This health-related and illness-related perspective of disability is known as the medical model of disability. It assumes several things about the nature of disability (Box 1.4).

The philosophy of medicine has traditionally been to treat and to cure but in rehabilitation these outcomes are unlikely and the aim has been to normalize. This philosophy was reinforced by the initial classification of the WHO that produced a distinction between impairment, disability, and handicap. The medical model of disability usually implies that it is the physician who should take a leading role in the entire rehabilitation process—being team leader, organizing programmes of care, and generally directing the delivery of services for the disabled person. The doctor/patient relationship was the senior relationship in the medical model. Rehabilitation was born around the First World War when there was a very strong philosophy of the doctor telling injured servicemen how to behave, how to get better, and how to get back as quickly as possible to active duty. Such a model may have been appropriate in that cultural context but is now outdated. In recent years the central role of the physician has, in general, been subsumed by the central role of the multidisciplinary team. It is now realized that all health and social service professionals have their own role to play in the overall rehabilitation programme for the disabled person. However, even modern multidisciplinary rehabilitation is still largely based on the philosophy of the medical model—just a little watered down.

Box 1.4 Assumptions of the medical model of disability

- Disability is individualized. It is regarded as a disease state that is located within an individual. Thus, the problem and solution may both be found within that person.
- Disability is a disease state. A deviation from the norm. It inherently necessitates some form of treatment or cure.
- Being disabled, a person is regarded inherently as biologically or psychologically inferior to that of the able-bodied and normal human being.
- Disability is viewed as a personal tragedy. It assumes the presence of a victim. The objective normality state that is assumed by professionals gives them a dominant decision-making role often noted in a typical doctor/patient relationship.

After Laing R (1998). A critique of the disability movement. *Asia Pacific Disability and Rehabilitation Journal* **9**, 4–8.

Social model of disability

Disability lobby groups have long suggested that the fundamental construct of disability is that a person's impairment is not the cause of their restriction of activity but rather it is the organization of society that discriminates against them. The social model focuses on the fact that disability is a construction of society and if society could accept and accommodate disabled people, both physically and attitudinally, then disability as a concept would be made redundant. The key features of the social model are listed in Box 1.5.

As the disability movement developed, particularly in the United States after the Vietnam War and in the UK in the 1980s, there was a feeling of antagonism between health professionals involved in disability on the one hand and activists in the disability movement on the other hand. There was limited cooperation. These two extreme positions have now rather softened and disabled people realize that health professionals have a clear and important role in helping to minimize activity restrictions. This is particularly true in the post-acute setting after, for example, stroke or traumatic brain injury. Even in longer-term disability, such as cerebral palsy or multiple sclerosis (MS), the health professional still has a key role to play. The crude dichotomy between the medical model and the social model is slowly but surely being replaced by a more appropriate halfway house—which could be called the *partnership model of disability*.

Box 1.5 Assumptions of the social model of disability

- A person's impairment is not the cause of restriction of activity.
- The cause of restriction is the organization of society.
- Society discriminates against disabled people.
- Attitudinal, sensory, architectural, and economic barriers are of equal, if not greater, importance than health barriers.
- Less emphasis is placed on the involvement of health professionals in the life of the disabled person.

Terminology

In the disability literature and in clinical practice it is vital to use correct terminology. This is not mere political correctness. Incorrect terminology can not only be demeaning but can indicate an inappropriate philosophy or attitude from the individual concerned or indeed from the whole multi-disciplinary team.

It is important to avoid terminology that implies dependency or termi-nology which just categorizes all disabled people. The word 'patient', for example, may be entirely appropriate for someone who is acutely ill and in the short term dependent upon medical and health professionals. However, in rehabilitation, if one agrees with the philosophy underlying the social model of disability, then disabled people are not ill and thus 'patient' is not a term that is appropriate. When the rehabilitation process is striving to give that person independence and develop new skills then terminology that implies the opposite should be avoided. There are a number of other group classifications that must be avoided including:
• Epileptics
• Stroke sufferers
• MS sufferers
• Spastics
• Young chronic sick
• The handicapped
• The disabled.

Although there is no universally accepted terminology it does seem rea-sonable to use the term 'disabled person' or 'person with a disability'. Correct terminology simply means that the person is being treated as an individual and not simply labelled as an example of a particular group.

As with many sections of society, it does seem acceptable for the group members themselves to use self-derogatory terms. People with spinal cord injuries will often refer to themselves as 'paras' or 'tetras' or even 'crips'.

Disability terminology is a minefield waiting to trap the unwary. The strength of feeling on these issues should not be underestimated.

Approaches to rehabilitation

Rehabilitation can be defined as an active and dynamic process by which a disabled person is helped to acquire knowledge and skills in order to maximize physical, psychological, and social function. It is a process that maximizes functional ability and minimizes disability and handicap—thus promoting activity and participation. There are three basic approaches in rehabilitation:

- Approaches to reduce the limitations on activity.
- Approaches designed to acquire new skills and strategies, which will reduce the impact of the limitations to activity.
- Approaches that help to alter the environment, both the physical environment and the social environment, so that a given activity limitation carries with it as little problem in participation as possible.

These are three vital concepts to the understanding of the rehabilitation process. The following is an example of these three approaches in action.

Case example

A middle-aged man has MS. He has been working quite successfully in the post room of a large factory. He is married with two children and has an active social life. However, in recent months he has developed increasing problems with walking secondary to developing paraparesis complicated by spasticity. In addition he has recently developed difficulties with urinary frequency and urgency. Rehabilitation, using our three basic approaches, could be structured as follows:

- Attempts could be made to reduce his activity limitation by appropriate treatment of his spasticity and use of medication to control his bladder symptoms.
- He could learn new skills. He could learn, for example, to walk with external support such as a stick or even use a wheelchair for longer distances such as from the office car park to his place of work. He could be taught intermittent self-catheterization to assist his urinary problems.
- Approaches could be made to alter his work environment. He may, for example, be advised on the use of a perching stool so he can support himself whilst sorting the post. He may need to approach his employer to change or reduce his hours if prolonged periods of standing are leading to increasing fatigue. At home there may be a need to provide grab rails in the toilet or other adaptations to the bathroom or kitchen. His wife and family will clearly need to be involved in order to understand his condition and adjust the family lifestyle to cope with his new problems. His wife may begin to share the driving if problems of spasticity are beginning to interfere with his driving abilities over long distances.

Thus, there are many simple pointers that could help him to minimize the impact of his condition on his work, on his family, and on his leisure time. The rehabilitation team needs to keep in mind these three basic approaches when planning the rehabilitation programme.

Goal setting

The essence of rehabilitation is goal setting. The first goal to be established is the final strategic aim. This can vary significantly. For some a long-term goal would be returning to a completely normal lifestyle. For others it may simply be to return home and remain at home with the help of carers. In other cases it may be to take up part-time employment or resume a particular leisure interest. Sometimes much discussion, and even argument, is necessary in order that all parties can agree a realistic long-distance strategic goal. After such a goal has been established then steps need to be identified in order to achieve that goal. If, for example, a long-term goal is to be independently mobile without the use of aids then achieving that goal can be broken down into a number of shorter-term subgoals. This may, for example, start with sitting without support, then standing without support, then walking with assistance, then walking with aids, and finally independent walking over increasing distances. It is important to emphasize that the goals must be precise. It is inappropriate, for example, to set a goal such as to walk with an improved gait. This is not specific or measurable and is obviously open to considerable subjective interpretation. A better subgoal would be to walk 20 metres with the aid of a stick within a period of 30 seconds. Thus, goals need to be both specific and measurable. They also need to be achievable within the context of the underlying natural history or pathophysiology of the condition. In order for progress to be seen it is also useful for goals to be time limited. In a post-acute rehabilitation setting it is useful to plan for achievable subgoals in a period of 1 or perhaps 2 weeks whereas in people with longer-term disabilities such goals could be set over a much longer timescale. Finally each goal must be relevant for that individual. It may be relevant for some people to learn how to make a cup of tea but for others it may be more relevant to learn how to open a can of lager!

In summary, it is useful to remember the mnemonic SMART when goals are being met. All goals should be:
- **S**pecific
- **M**easurable
- **A**chievable
- **R**elevant
- **T**ime limited.

Outcome measurement

The disabled person and the rehabilitation team need to know when the goals have been achieved. It is important for each goal to have a valid and reliable outcome measure attached to it. A number of specific outcome measures are discussed later in this handbook. In summary, there are a number of measures that have been designed to monitor overall disability and/or quality of life that are useful for assessing progress towards longer-term goals. Shorter-term subgoals often need more specific outcome measures. Such examples would be specific measures of mobility, such as timed walking speed, specific measures of hand function, such as the Action Research Arm Test, or more specific psychological parameters, such as an objective measure of memory. Any outcome measure used needs to be specific to the outcome it is measuring as well as being both valid and reliable. There is little point in using an outcome measure that has not been validated and shown to be reliable for the particular circumstances in which it is used. This would be like measuring cooking ingredients on scales with the wrong weights. However, the scales need not, and indeed preferably should not, be complicated or time-consuming. Whilst specific and somewhat complicated measures of mobility are sometimes useful, particularly in a research setting, simple day-to-day, but objectively measurable, goals can also be used in a busy clinical situation. The ability to hold a saucepan with a given volume of water for a particular period of time is an example of a simple and objective goal that may be of practical relevance to that individual.

Whilst objectively measurable goals are useful it should obviously not be forgotten that the opinion of the disabled person and/or their family is of primary importance and should always be able to colour and adjust any objective measure. Objective measurement, whilst vital, should not be allowed to override the opinions, perceptions, and wishes of the disabled person. Indeed the disabled person should be the central figure in the setting of goals and their appropriate measurement and monitoring.

Benefits of rehabilitation

The specific benefits of rehabilitation will become self-evident in the later sections of this book. However, in general terms the benefits of rehabilitation can be summarized as follows:

Functional benefit

There is now significant evidence that a coordinated interdisciplinary rehabilitation approach can produce better functional outcome than traditional unidisciplinary service delivery. In terms of stroke, for example, a rehabilitation unit will produce more functional gain, more quickly, with a better chance of returning home and with decreased morbidity and mortality. There is a similar case in the context of traumatic brain injury. There is even now evidence of a functional benefit of rehabilitation in deteriorating conditions, such as MS. These specific issues are discussed in later sections. There is also now evidence that short-term gains in a rehabilitation unit can generalize into longer-term functional improvements. If longer contact with the rehabilitation team is not established then the short-term functional gains and new skills may fade with time. This emphasizes the importance of not only post-acute rehabilitation units but also longer-term community support as well as rehabilitation support for those with deteriorating problems. What is not known is which elements of the rehabilitation process produce such functional benefits. Is it the basic rehabilitation process or is it simply the multidisciplinary or interdisciplinary team—or both combined? There is room for much more research on this subject but it is very likely that it is the whole rehabilitation process outlined in preceding sections that is key to such functional benefit.

Reduction of unnecessary complications

The disabled person can easily run into unnecessary and additional problems as a result of unrecognized or untreated complications. Untreated spasticity, for example, can lead to muscle contracture which further worsens functionality, increases dependency, and places the person at a risk of even more complications, such as pressure sores. Other significant problems can arise, for example, with inappropriately treated incontinence or unrecognized depression. The following sections in the book will outline many such examples.

Better coordination and use of resources

The person with complex and severe disabilities needs a variety of health, social, and other services. There is the clear potential for unnecessary overlap of assessment, treatment, and follow-up. The rehabilitation team should act as a single point of contact and a single point of information for the disabled person and their family. The team should be in the best position to coordinate the various services. Many people with complex disabilities now have the benefit of a case manager whose key role is to coordinate the different health and social inputs. Ideally the disabled person or a key family member should act in this role but this is not always possible, particularly for those people with residual cognitive or intellectual challenges.

Cost-effective use of resources

Unfortunately there are few studies that confirm the cost benefits of rehabilitation. There are some studies which, in general, have shown such benefits. In Newcastle upon Tyne in the UK, for example, a multidisciplinary MS team was established in the city. The economic benefits, in terms of reduced hospital bed usage and reduced outpatient visits, were offset by the cost of the team itself so that the whole team was introduced as a cost-neutral venture. It seems self-evident, although research is still needed, that better functional gains and avoidance of unnecessary complications should make the best use of scarce health and social resources. If a disabled person can be assisted back to work, even on a part-time basis, then it is a major cost saving for the national economy. About 80% of the costs of disability are due to lost employment opportunities.

Education, training, and research

There is a need for further studies in the whole realm of rehabilitation. Much more education, training, and research is needed. A rehabilitation team can act in such an education and research capacity and can help to enhance knowledge, reduce ignorance, and go some way to reducing the discrimination in disability.

Summary

This introductory chapter has outlined the concepts, principles, and processes of rehabilitation and illustrated some of the benefits. It is a process of education and enablement that centrally involves the disabled person and their family. It is a process that must be conducted through a series of specific goals on route to a long-term strategic aim. We now know that rehabilitation can produce real benefit in terms of functional improvement, fewer unnecessary complications, better coordination of services, and cost-effectiveness as well as providing a key role in general education, training, and research for both professionals and disabled people.

In summary the basic tasks of rehabilitation are:
- To work in partnership with the disabled person and their family.
- To give accurate information and advice about the nature of the disability, natural history, prognosis, etc.
- To listen to the needs and perceptions of the disabled person and their family.
- To assist in the establishment of realistic rehabilitation goals appropriate to that person's disability, family, social, and employment needs.
- To establish appropriate measures so that the disabled person and the rehabilitation team know when such goals have been obtained.
- To work with all colleagues in an interdisciplinary fashion.
- To liaise as needed with carers and advocates of the disabled person.
- To foster appropriate education and training of health and social service professionals as well as helping to meet the educational requirements of the disabled person.
- To foster research, both quantitative and qualitative, into the many aspects of the rehabilitation service—from scientific principles to the basic service delivery.

Rehabilitation has in the past been viewed as a rather vague and woolly process—often with justification. However, modern rehabilitation should be a combination of a precise science and the art of traditional medicine.

Further reading

1. Brisenden S (1986). Independent living in the medical model. *Disability, Handicap and Society* **1**, 173–8.
2. Dobkin BH (ed.) (2003). *The Clinical Science of Neurologic Rehabilitation*, 2nd edn. Oxford University Press, Oxford.
3. Greenwood RJ, Barnes MP, MacMillan M, *et al.* (eds) (2003). *Handbook of Neurological Rehabilitation*. Psychology Press, Hove.
4. Shakespeare T (2006). *Disability rights and wrongs*. Routledge, Oxford.
5. Wade DT (ed.) (1996). *Measurement in Neurological Rehabilitation*. Oxford University Press, Oxford.
6. ⌂ www.direct.gov.uk/en/DisabledPeople—a useful generic website produced by the UK government.
7. ⌂ www.disabilityresources.org—a very useful website that provides access to many hundreds of resources on the web regarding disability issues.
8. ⌂ www.who.int/classifications/icf

Epidemiology

Introduction

Epidemiology is the study of patterns of disease occurrence in populations and of factors that influence these patterns. Knowledge of epidemiology is linked with the natural history of a disease or condition, and is therefore relevant to clinical practice. It is also relevant to Rehabilitation Medicine, as it categorizes how people with disabilities function.

Incidence and prevalence of a condition

- *Incidence*: number of new cases appearing in a unit time, e.g. per year.
- *Prevalence*: number of affected people in a population at any one time. (7.8 million people with a disability in UK)
- Differences between the two may be small or large depending on the survival of patients.
- Conditions with a high prevalence may have a significant impact on resource allocation, e.g. osteoarthritis, stroke, traumatic brain injury.
- Rapidly progressive problems, e.g. cancers and motor neuron disease demand rapid and flexible responses in the knowledge that service provision may require change after only a short time.
- Rehabilitation services are more concerned with prevalence than with incidence.

Disability is common with 14% of the adult population of the UK having a disability (Table 2.1). The prevalence of disability among adults aged 16 years and over was 135 per 1000 population and, if one includes those people living in institutions, the prevalence increases to 142 per 1000. 77% of disabled people were found to have one or more of these physical disabilities, implying a prevalence rate of 104.1 per 1000 aged 16 years and over, living in the community, and 109 per 1000, including those living in institutions. Although locomotion disability is the most common for all age groups the combination of physical and mental disabilities, appears to be the most disabling.

Table 2.1 Disability domains—estimates of prevalence of disability in Great Britain by type (ICIDH) and age

Type of disability	Age group			
	16–59	60–74	75+	All adults
Locomotion	31	198	496	99
Hearing	17	110	328	59
Personal care	18	99	313	57
Dexterity	13	78	199	40
Seeing	9	56	262	38
Intellectual function	20	40	109	34
Behaviour	19	40	152	31
Reaching and stretching	9	54	149	28
Communication	12	42	140	27
Continence	9	42	147	26
Disfigurement	5	18	27	9
Eating, drinking, and digesting	2	12	30	6
Consciousness	5	10	9	5

Reproduced with permission from Martin J, Meltzer H, and Elliot D (1988). *OPCS Report 1, The Prevalence of Disability Among Adults*. HMSO, London.

International Classification of Functioning, Disability and Health (ICF)

The WHO published the International Classification of Impairments, Disability and Handicap (ICIDH) in 1980 as part of its preparation for the International Year for the Disabled in 1981. This was widely adopted in clinical practice and became established as a means to initiate the rehabilitation process. However, over the ensuing years, its shortcomings became apparent, particularly when disabled people were clinically managed in different settings. In addition, it was seen as negative and highlighted a person's dependence. As a result, a further classification was produced in 1997, in which the disability and handicap domains were replaced by the more positive 'activity' and 'participation' terms. This still did not go far enough in recognizing the impact of disability on a person's life and did not translate from health care to social aspects of life. The ICF was thus established in 2001 and attempts to add personal and environmental factors, which have an important role in the perception of limitations to functioning and participation. It recognizes the impact of a health condition on a person's functioning in terms of loss of organ functioning and thus functioning, but also associates this with loss of personal functioning and participation limitation. Just because a person has am impairment, e.g. a foot drop, it does not mean that he or she is limited in activities and in participation. It depends on the context of a person's life and on the surrounding environment. For instance, this impairment may only have little impact on the participation of a middle-aged professional person working in an office, but would probably be profoundly limiting on a manual worker or a professional sportsman.

The WHO published its International Classification of Functioning and Health in 2001.[1] This has been fundamental to the better analysis of the consequences of disease and to the practice of Rehabilitation Medicine. It highlights the differences between the medical or from the rehabilitation perspective of the impact of a disease on an individual. From the medical or disease perspective, patients' functioning, disability, and health are seen primarily as the consequences or the impact of a disease or health condition. Medical interventions are targeted towards the disease process and the ultimate goal of these interventions is to avoid the consequences on the individual. From the rehabilitation perspective, patients' functioning and health are seen as associated with and not merely a consequence of a health condition or disease. Functioning represents not only an outcome, but also the starting point of the clinical assessment and intervention. It has a close interaction with the person's characteristics and environment. Thus, the rehabilitative process targets functioning, the environment, and modifiable personal factors. Rehabilitation, therefore, begins with an in-depth understanding of the determinants of functioning and of its interactions with personal and environmental factors regardless of the health condition (Figs. 2.1 and 2.2).

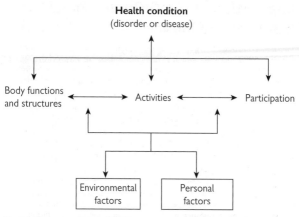

Fig. 2.1 The current framework of functioning and disability—the WHO International Classification of Functioning, Disability and Health (ICF). Reproduced from International Classification of Functioning, Disability and Health (ICF) ⌕ www. who.int/classifications/icf WHO press© with permission.

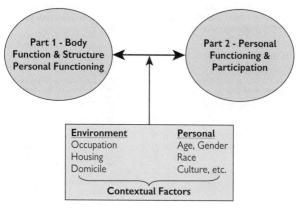

Fig. 2.2 ICF as applied to Rehabilitation Medicine

References

1. WHO (2001). International classification of functioning, disability and health WHO, Geneva. ⌕ www.who.int/classifications/icf

Application of the Office for Population, Censuses and Surveys*

There has not been a major survey of disability in the UK since that of the OPCS in 1988 and 1989, which gave a comprehensive view on the lives of disabled people. It also attempted to produce a tool, whereby the impact of disability could be measured in terms of personal functioning and participation in daily life, but this has not been widely adopted.

In the UK most disability is due to musculoskeletal disease and is followed by problems related to the eye and ear. Generally speaking, neurological conditions make up a smaller component, but have far greater relevance in the more severe categories of disability on the OPCS. scale. In fact, severe disability in younger people is primarily due to neurological disease.

Severe disability is also associated with multiple pathology and people >60 years of age are more likely to have two or more conditions, which increase with age. Arthritis and hypertension, the two conditions with the highest prevalence, co-existed in over one quarter of those aged 60 years and over. Because of this association with co-morbid disease, there exists an essential difference between the rehabilitation of older people compared to younger groups. Certain conditions are more prevalent in different parts of the country—e.g. MS increases as one moves north throughout the UK—and services have to reflect the needs of local populations. In addition, the affluence and social circumstances of certain parts of the UK appears to be reflected by a concomitant change in the levels of disability and disadvantage and this is perhaps based on occupational and different levels of educational attainment and income.

Table 2.2 OPCS classification by type and severity of disability[1]

Type of disability	Severity %					
	1–2	3–4	5–6	7–8	9–10	Total
Other disability (not physical)	38	26	17	5	0	23
Physical	39	35	31	25	18	33
Physical and sensory	21	31	30	36	28	28
Physical and mental (± sensory)	2	8	24	34	56	18
Total	100	100	100	100	100	100

1. Reproduced with permission from Martin J, Meltzer H, and Elliott D (1989). *OPCS Report 4, Disabled Adults, Services, Transport and Employment*. HMSO, London.

*Now known as Office for National Statistics.

Table 2.3 Frequency of disease groups causing physical disabilities and all disability—adults in private households.[1]

Disease ICD Group	Type of disability				
	All Types	Locomotor	Reaching and stretching	Dexterity	Disfigurement
Musculoskeletal	46	56	64	67	6
Ear	38	1	0	0	1
Eye	22	2	0	1	2
Circulatory	20	23	10	7	5
Mental	13	3	2	3	1
Nervous system	13	12	21	22	12
Respiratory	13	14	3	2	1
Digestive	6	2	2	1	5
Genitourinary	3	1	1	0	2
Neoplasms	2	1	3	2	4
Endocrine	2	2	1	1	1
Infections	1	1	1	1	3
Blood	1	0	0	0	0
Skin	1	1	0	0	4
Congenital	0	0	0	0	3
Other	6	5	3	4	1

1. Reproduced with permission from Martin J, Meltzer H, and Elliott D (1989). *OPCS Report 4, Disabled Adults, Services, Transport and Employment.* HMSO, London.

How does epidemiological information help us?

It is important in Rehabilitation Medicine to know whether one is trying to change a person's impairment, functioning, or participation. For instance, if the goal of rehabilitation is to allow a person with impaired mobility to get upstairs and use the bathroom, one could approach the problem in three ways.

- Definitive treatment could be directed at the pathology and impairment to diminish their effects and restore function in the limbs.
- Functioning could be addressed with the result that, despite a continuing impairment, the person could be trained to climb the stairs and walk to the bathroom.
- A chair lift and a wheelchair could be provided, such that he or she could be transported upstairs, transferred to a wheelchair at the top of the stairs and then be either taken or take themselves to the bathroom.

Although the ultimate aim would be the same, the options would involve different activities by different people at different levels and with a different impact on the disabled person and their family.

Participation is quite the most difficult domain to address as it varies from person to person according to their circumstances and is often outside the control of the health-based rehabilitation team. A disabled person's life satisfaction is the most difficult to measure, as reduced participation is not an inevitable and direct consequence of impairment and disability. It actually arises from an interaction of the impairment and functioning with other external factors, such as the home environment, the job, personal relations etc. Its impact derives from society's general attitude to disabled people and it is influenced by culture and by society's values and expectations. For instance, the expectations of the parents of disabled adolescents are significantly lower where there is a congenital disability (or one from a very early age) compared to an acquired disability. The impact of a physical disability on the life of an individual is therefore not just related to the disease process or to the number of individual disabilities, but to what are termed as contextual factors. These include:

- Orientation
- Physical independence
- Mobility
- Occupation
- Social integration
- Economic self-sufficiency.

Badley's model (1991)[1] encapsulates these factors (Fig. 2.3). Many people can be severely affected by disability, but are quite satisfied with their lifestyles, whereas others, with similar or lesser disabilities, may be unable to exist.

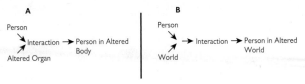

Fig. 2.3 Human experience of disablement

References

1. Badley EM and Tennant A (1991) A survey of disablement in a british population using an action oriented measure, physical independence handicap: problems with activities of daily living and level of support. *International disability studies* **13**(3), 91–98.

Chapter 3

The rehabilitation team

Rehabilitation teams

Rehabilitation is about team work. It is a process that has to involve a wide range of different professionals. Rehabilitation teams can work in many different contexts. Many teams will be hospital based and working primarily with people after a stroke or traumatic brain injury. Such teams will mainly involve physicians, therapists, and nurses. However, other teams can work in a different context and team membership will have a different emphasis. A community rehabilitation team is more likely to involve local authority employees, such as social workers and community occupational therapists, and perhaps other professionals, such as employment experts. Thus, it is not possible, or indeed desirable, to define disciplines that must be members of a rehabilitation team. Indeed a list of such disciplines will inappropriately emphasize professional boundaries.

The essence of the rehabilitation team is that it is not simply a collection of different professionals but a coherent group of such professionals working together for the common good of the disabled person. A simple collection of appropriate professionals could be called a *multidisciplinary team*. Whilst such a team may contain the necessary range of professionals, evidence shows that such a team does not produce the necessary benefits that should flow from the rehabilitation process. The rehabilitation team must function as a coherent whole so that client-centred goals can be set and monitored and such goals should cross traditional professional boundaries. The team should not be *discipline orientated but outcome orientated*.

There is extensive literature on the definition of teams but the following list (after Furnell et al.[1]) provides a useful summary of the main characteristics of a rehabilitation team:

- Professionals from different disciplines who meet regularly.
- The allocation, by each member, of a significant proportion of his/her own time to the pursuit of a team's objectives.
- Agreement on explicit objectives for the team that determine the team's structure and function.
- Adequate administrative and clinical coordination to support the work of the team, although not necessarily by the same person on all occasions.
- A defined geographical base.
- A clear differentiation of and respect for those skills and roles that are specific and unique to individual members as well as recognition of those roles that may be shared.

References

1. Furnell J, Flett S, and Clarke DF (1987). Multidisciplinary clinical teams: some issues in establishment and function. *Hospital and Health Services Review*, January, 15–18.

Why have teams?

There is evidence that a proper rehabilitation team can produce functional benefit for the disabled person over and above a collection of individuals working together as a group. Some of the benefits of such team work are likely to be:

- Improved communication.
- Sharing of knowledge between people of different disciplines.
- A more consistent goal-orientated approach and better continuity of care.
- Promotion of a broad perspective for rehabilitation provision.
- Provision of a stimulating environment to enhance the contribution of team members, improve motivation, and increase individual effectiveness.
- Creation of an 'esprit de corps' that leads to a mutually supporting atmosphere.

These characteristics are useful as they emphasize not only the importance of the rehabilitation team for the disabled person but also the importance of the team for its constituent members. Rehabilitation is a broad subject and no individual can carry all the necessary knowledge and information required to provide a cohesive and thorough rehabilitation programme. Single practitioners working by themselves, often in the community, can begin to feel lonely and isolated and part of a team function is mutual support, recognition of problems, and development of a team culture where no one individual feels isolated or overwhelmed.

Further reading

1. Wood RL (2003). The rehabilitation team. In: *Handbook of Neurological Rehabilitation*, 2nd edn (ed. Greenwood RJ, Barnes MP, McMillan TM, and Ward CD), pp.41–50. Psychology Press, Hove.

Interdisciplinary teams

The essence of rehabilitation is the focusing of goal setting and the needs of a particular individual with a disability. Individuals rarely package their particular requirements into neat professional boundaries. An individual will rarely say that he or she has a specific physiotherapy goal, an occupational therapy goal, or a clinical psychology goal. The individual's goals are most likely to cross professional boundaries. A rehabilitation team must recognize the importance of such client-centred goals and adjust their own work patterns accordingly. If, for example, a long-term goal is to walk independently then an appropriate subgoal may be to sit to stand and transfer independently. The physiotherapist is likely to be the key team member that works with the disabled person in achieving this goal. However, it is still the responsibility of the other team members to heed the advice of the physiotherapist and work with the client to achieve that particular aim. The speech and language therapist carrying out their session will need to be aware of how the patient stands up and moves from one chair to another in the room, just as much as the physiotherapist will need to be aware of the communication strategy that might be led by the speech and language therapist.

This approach is termed *interdisciplinary working*. The members of the rehabilitation team will need to flexible and prepared to work across artificial professional boundaries. 'That's not my job' is not an attitude required in a rehabilitation team. Interdisciplinary working implies a blurring of professional roles whilst still preserving the separate identity and expertise of individual professions. The ultimate goal of this approach is to produce an integrated assessment and to develop a unified treatment plan that is jointly carried out by all team members. Thus, it demands a higher degree of group interaction and focused treatment effort than a simple multidisciplinary team. It is also a team that should incorporate the disabled person and their family as part of the team itself. It is equally important for family members to understand the goals and the methods by which they are being achieved. Such understanding can only come if the family is an integral part of the rehabilitation team.

Further reading

1. Abreu BC, Zhang L, Seale G, *et al.* (2002) Interdisciplinary meetings: investigating the collaboration between persons with brain injury and treatment teams. *Brain Injury*, **16**(8), 691–704.

Generic rehabilitation workers

This is a concept in rehabilitation that is gathering momentum. The ultimate role extension must be to completely blur professional boundaries. Such therapists are no longer identified as physiotherapists, occupational therapists, or clinical psychologists but simply co-partners in a rehabilitation team. This ultimate approach implies a broad-based generic training which currently does not exist (except perhaps in the somewhat artificial environment of conductive education as practised in the Peto Institute in Budapest and other centres). This is probably a model that works better in the context of the rehabilitation of neurobehavioural problems after traumatic brain injury. This type of rehabilitation, especially in the later stages of recovery, requires a particular emphasis on communication and coordination of care so that the individual has a coordinated, well-documented, and consistent response to various behavioural problems.

The members of such a team, often led by a clinical neuropsychologist, work in a *transdisciplinary* fashion where professional boundaries are no longer recognized. However, the neurobehavioural team is a specific example and it may be very difficult, and perhaps inappropriate, to apply this in a more traditional post-acute rehabilitation unit. Nevertheless, in such units most of the day-to-day rehabilitation can be carried out by *generic health-care workers* who work under the guidance of the qualified therapist. These generic assistants often take on the role of a keyworker and are the main point of contact between the disabled person and a broader-based team. There are many different models. In some centres such an assistant takes on an important coordinating and educational role for the disabled person whilst in other centres the assistant is more subsidiary to the qualified therapist. Regrettably there is little research that enables meaningful comparisons to be made between different models of rehabilitation team working.

Keyworker or case manager

Whatever model of working is adopted by the rehabilitation team there are always a large number of individuals who need to liaise with the disabled person. This can produce a sense of confusion or a lack of direction. Teams have developed different ways around this problem. A common system is the allocation of a *keyworker*. One team member is allocated to be the key liaison between the team, the disabled person, and the family. The keyworker acts as the main source of information about the rehabilitation process and feeds back the thoughts and aspirations of the disabled person to the team, and vice versa. This system should not be seen as a substitute for regular team meetings nor should there be an abrogation of responsibility by relevant professionals. It is simply part of the whole rehabilitation team process that may lead to better coordination and liaison and clear channels of communication.

In theory the keyworker can be any team member as long as that individual has an appropriate range of interpersonal skills and broad background knowledge of the needs and requirements of the disabled person. In many cases it would be entirely appropriate for the disabled person him/herself to act as the keyworker. However, this is not always possible, particularly if the person has troublesome cognitive and intellectual problems. If an advocate is required it is probably inappropriate for the advocate to act as the keyworker. The role of the advocate is purely to advocate the cause of the disabled person whereas the role of a keyworker is often one of negotiation and arbitration when opinions and goals diverge or are felt to be unrealistic.

In some cases the role of the keyworker can be extended to that of a *case manager*. The concept of case management has been developed as a way of assisting disabled people with the coordination of the necessary professional staff. Case management can include:
- Simple coordination within a single agency.
- Coordination across agency boundaries.
- Service brokerage in which the case manager negotiates with the key agencies on the client's behalf.
- Budget-holding responsibility where services can be purchased on behalf of the client from statutory bodies or other voluntary and private agencies.

Although there have been few controlled studies of the efficacy of case management it is now a widely practised role and almost certainly provides a better and more coherent service and assists people, particularly those with cognitive impairment, to find their way through the maze of services. Indeed the role of case manager is now being seen as a separate and valid profession and care must be taken to ensure that a professional role designed to reduce and cross professional boundaries does not in itself produce a new professional discipline!

Core team

Despite the importance of interdisciplinary working there is still a core membership for a health-orientated rehabilitation team. Core members of the team are:
- Rehabilitation nurse
- Clinical neuropsychologist
- Occupational therapist
- Physiotherapist
- Speech and language therapist
- Rehabilitation physician.

It is difficult to envisage a post-acute rehabilitation team that does not have access to such individuals. However, the team will often need to draw on a wide range of other expertise, such as social work and counselling, as well as having occasional access to dieticians, chiropodists, and rehabilitation engineers. Sometimes access to other medical specialties is required, such as urology and orthopaedic surgery. In the community there often needs to be a broader network of core individuals. Health requirements quickly change to social requirements and input from social service occupational therapists and social workers soon becomes crucial. At later stages useful links can be fostered with employment rehabilitation experts as well as other voluntary providers, lawyers, social security staff, and a variety of disability support groups.

Thus, there is the concept of a *nuclear team* and the *support team*. The former comprises those people most involved with the individual on a day-to-day basis. The support team are more peripherally involved. The support team are usually not so 'hands on' and may not be in daily contact with either the disabled individual or the team. They could be said to act as consultants to the team rather than being intrinsic team members.

Team leadership

This can be a problem. The leader of many rehabilitation teams is the physician. This is usually for historical or political reasons and not necessarily because the doctor makes the best leader. Indeed it can be argued that medical training by its very nature encourages autonomous independent thinking in order to make quick decisions in acute situations and that this style is not best suited to the qualities required of a team leader. However, it has to be recognized that in many organizations, and in many cultures, it is not practical to suggest that anyone other than the doctor should lead the team. There are some advantages that medicine has over other specialisms. Medical training is able to give a broad overview of a particular disorder rather than the potentially narrower perspective of other professional disciplines. The doctor should be able to have a view of the 'whole person' with some grasp of the role of other professionals, and an understanding of the complementary role of team members can be a useful characteristic. However, the team leader needs to have other qualities. A leader has usefully been described as someone tolerant enough to listen to others but strong enough to reject their advice. The other characteristics that need to be displayed by a leader include:

- Good interpersonal and social skills.
- Vision for the long-term future of the team.
- Communication skills.
- Listening skills.
- Flexibility—the ability to listen to others and adjust the direction of the team according to the thoughts and views of other team members.
- Toughness—to make difficult decisions as and when they arise.
- Organizational skills.
- Good time management—to devote enough time to the team activities rather than just clinical tasks.
- Financial and budgetary understanding.
- Political skills—to influence colleagues and managers and direct maximum resources to the team.

It is doubtful whether such an individual exists who can fulfil all these criteria!

Whilst hospital-based teams are still usually under the direction of the hospital consultant there are now an increasing number of teams with non-medical team leaders, particularly in a community setting, or teams with an emphasis on the neurobehavioural and cognitive problems of disabled people.

Overall there is no doubt that the right leader is more important than their professional background.

Organization of services

Principles of service delivery

This section will look at the various organizational aspects of the delivery of a comprehensive rehabilitation service. There is no single way to develop a rehabilitation service and the physical base, team, structure, and scope and range of the services provided will clearly vary from community to community. This chapter will outline some of the possibilities for the organization of services and discuss the merits and drawbacks of different systems.

However, no matter how the team is structured it should first establish the basic principles under which it chooses to work. A useful set of principles was produced by the Prince of Wales Advisory Group on Disability (now The Disability Partnership) in 1985.[1] These are as follows:

• Disabled people and their family should be consulted as services are planned.
• Information should be clearly presented and readily available to all disabled consumers.
• The life of disabled people in the local and national community should be promoted with respect to both responsibilities and benefits.
• Disabled people should have a choice as to where to live and how to maintain independence, including help in learning how to choose.
• There should be recognition that long-term disability is not synonymous with illness and that the medical model of care is inappropriate in the majority of cases.
• The service should provide autonomy for the freedom to make decisions regarding a way of life best suited to an individual disabled person's circumstances.

Although not part of the Prince of Wales' principles a seventh principle could be added:

• A fully comprehensive range of rehabilitation services should be provided as close to an individual's home as possible.

Most comprehensive rehabilitation systems are based on a two-tier service. Most rehabilitation can and should be carried out either at home or in the individual's own neighbourhood. Thus, each community should have an accessible and local rehabilitation team. However, it also has to be recognized that some disabled people, probably around 10%, will require the expertise and facilities of a more specialist service. Hopefully some elements of a specialist service can be delivered locally but almost certainly there will need to be a regional specialist rehabilitation centre to complement and supplement the services provided by the local team.

The range and type of services required at a regional level and at a local level will obviously depend on the availability of appropriately trained staff, resources, and facilities and will vary from area to area. Close links between the regional services and the local services are vital. The disabled client should be able to move seamlessly from one service to the other with continuity of care, and preferably a local therapist should remain in touch with the client whilst the individual is within the regional centre and vice versa. However, resources are scarce and an ideal, fully interlinked, two-tier rehabilitation system is difficult to achieve.

References

1. Prince of Wales' Advisory Group on Disability (1985). *Living options: guidelines for those planning services for people with severe physical disabilities.* Prince of Wales' Advisory Group on Disability, London.

Regional rehabilitation services

The regional specialist rehabilitation centre should work on the same underlying philosophy as any local team. It should work on the same principles of rehabilitation, particularly interdisciplinary team work, goal setting, and properly documented outcome measures. The regional team will consist of more specialist therapists, physicians, and nurses and will probably contain a more specialist range of equipment and assessment facilities. The population served by each centre will vary considerably according to the range and scope of the local team, of the local geography, and of the local resources. However, the following list of services should be provided from a regional centre as the skills or equipment required are unlikely to be available locally:

- A specialist rehabilitation service for people with the most complex multiple disabilities, particularly those with traumatic brain injury who have a combination of physical, psychological, and behavioural problems.
- A spinal injury service—in the UK there is a network of separate spinal injury regional centres, which developed historically under the original guidance of Sir Ludwig Guttman of Stoke Mandeville Hospital.
- A specialist service for complex wheelchair and special seating needs.
- A regional bioengineering service.
- A communication aids centre to provide specialist equipment for those with the most complicated communication problems.
- A centre for advice and assessment on assistive technology, particularly environmental control systems.
- An information, advice, and assessment service for car driving for disabled people.
- A service for amputees and adults and children with limb deformities (such as brachial plexus injuries, traumatic amputation, etc.).
- An inpatient service for assessment and perhaps long-term care of people in prolonged coma, prolonged vegetative state, or a minimally conscious state.
- A range of specialist outpatient services that are not provided more locally. The range of outpatient support will vary considerably but potential services are likely to include the following:
  - Spasticity clinic.
  - Botulinum toxin injection service for spasticity and other conditions such as dystonia.
  - A sexual counselling and advice service for disabled people.
  - A specialist orthotic service.
  - Specialist neuropsychological clinics, particularly for those with cognitive, intellectual, and memory problems.
  - A specialist neurobehavioural service (both inpatient and outpatient), particularly for people with behavioural problems in the context of traumatic brain injury.

The regional centre should also be a focus for education and training for health professionals, both within the centre and for the local teams, and indeed other health and social services professionals around the region. Thus, lecture facilities and appropriate libraries and other Internet resources should be provided. Finally the regional centre could also act as a focus for rehabilitation research and a link with a local academic centre would be important.

The design of the regional centre is also important. It should include realistic assessment areas such as kitchens, bathrooms, toilets, and bedrooms. It should certainly have a wide range of specialist equipment, such as specialist wheelchairs and assistive technology for assessment and demonstration purposes. Outdoor areas need to be provided for outdoor walking training, with different surfaces, and probably a car driving track would be necessary for the range of driving adaptation equipment to be properly demonstrated. If disabled people and their families are travelling a considerable distance then suitable overnight facilities or facilities for relatives to stay for a period of time would also be desirable.

Local rehabilitation services

The local rehabilitation team should be able to deliver all standard post-acute inpatient rehabilitation for individuals in the locality. Following a government mandate all district general hospitals in the UK who take acute admissions must now have a stroke rehabilitation unit. However, it is important that inpatient services for those with other post-acute rehabilitation requirements are not missed out, particularly for those people with more complex neurological problems such as moderate brain injury, multiple sclerosis, motor neuron disease, etc. An inpatient rehabilitation unit at a local level should clearly have close links, both clinical and educational, with a regional centre. A regional centre should be able to receive referrals from the local unit and once a particular problem has been successfully managed the individual should be sent back to the local inpatient unit and from there back into the community.

However, a local inpatient unit, whilst important, goes only a small way to meet all the health needs of disabled people in a locality. Most people after discharge from an inpatient unit will continue to have rehabilitation requirements. There are many disabled people who will never have an acute event (such as those with cerebral palsy, multiple sclerosis, etc.) and thus would never come into contact with a hospital-based post-acute rehabilitation unit. There is an obvious need for a community focused, and preferably community-based, rehabilitation team. The various models of such services are described later in this section.

In specific terms a local rehabilitation team should be able to provide all or most of the following:

- An inpatient post-acute rehabilitation service—particularly after stroke and moderate traumatic brain injury as well as occasional assessment and respite facilities for those with progressive conditions such as multiple sclerosis.
- A service for people with continence problems.
- A local orthotic service.
- A local prescription and maintenance service for basic wheelchairs.
- A nursing-based service for those with pressure sores.
- A counselling service that helps individuals with adjustment and coping problems in the context of physical disability—including sexual counselling.
- An appropriate range of outpatient support services.
- A rehabilitation liaison service with the acute medical, surgical, and psychiatric wards for those with physical disabilities who require other hospital admission.
- An aids and equipment service, probably including local provision of environmental control equipment.
- A basic information and advice service.

The local team will need to maintain a broad network of contacts with other relevant professionals and departments, including the local authority social service department, housing department, local employment rehabilitation service, and social security office. Local disability groups should also be associated with the local team and can provide invaluable peer support and information.

Rehabilitation unit

The rehabilitation team will need a physical base. There are many advantages to the creation of a dedicated rehabilitation unit. A physical unit is obviously required for a post-acute inpatient facility. However, even a community-based team will need a physical base to provide rooms for seeing clients, displaying equipment, and putting on seminars as well as providing necessary administrative support. Thus, every locality should have a clearly identified physical base. Ideally the rehabilitation unit needs to have the following facilities:

- An appropriate number of inpatient beds—the figure will vary considerably according to local needs and resources but around 20 beds would probably meet the post-acute rehabilitation needs of the 16–65-year-old population with (post-acute) neurological disabilities for a population of around 250 000 people.
- Communal living spaces.
- Practice kitchen, bedroom, and living areas.
- A self-contained flat to allow further practice at daily living skills for individuals about to return to the community.
- Space for appropriate outpatient clinics—although many services ought to be provided either in the home or even more local facilities, such as the GP surgery or other community centre.
- Space for information displays.
- Seminar and teaching space as well as meeting areas for the local team and perhaps local voluntary and disability groups.
- Plenty of appropriate car parking and ready access to accessible transport links.

The unit itself should obviously be fully accessible for people with a whole range of disabilities.

The presence of a physical unit is likely to be conducive to the development of an identifiable rehabilitation team, which should promote staff morale and stimulate education, training, and research. There are advantages if the unit is based separately from acute hospital wards. Moving to a separate rehabilitation unit can be seen as a step towards return to the community and might allow for more appropriate 'non-hospital' design.

Organizational models—the outpatient clinic

Equal delivery of health care to the disabled population is a major logistical task. As 14% of the adult population have a disability and at least 2–3% of the population have a severe disability then it is clear that a local rehabilitation service will need to see a large number of people—many of whom will need to be seen on an ongoing basis. There are many different models of service delivery and no single model is preferable to another. The service design must meet the local needs and take into account other local and regional resources, staffing, and facilities. Even in one area it is likely that several of the service models described in the next sections could apply.

The traditional model for short- and long-term support of people with disabilities is through the hospital outpatient clinic. The *advantages* of the outpatient service are:

- It is easier logistically to see people in one physical setting from the point of view of maximum use of staff time.
- It may be possible for the same inpatient team who looked after an individual in the post-acute setting to continue to see that individual on an outpatient basis—thus ensuring continuity of care.
- It may be possible to arrange outpatients so that individuals with the same sort of problem can attend for a particular clinic—for example, to provide a specific multiple sclerosis clinic or a Parkinson's disease clinic, or alternatively symptom-based clinics such as a continence clinic or a spasticity clinic. This service would enable an expert multidisciplinary team to be on hand at each clinic and provide the necessary assessment and treatment as well as providing appropriate information and advice. Such a clinic could act as a focus for the relevant local self-help group.

However, there are a number of significant *disadvantages* to an outpatient system:

- The outpatient clinics often run on a medical model with junior medical staff seeing the individual—often for the first time and with little prior knowledge of the disability or circumstances.
- There is little time to spend with each individual.
- Reappointment intervals tend to be several months apart when shorter intervals are sometimes more appropriate.
- It may be difficult to involve other relevant members of the multidisciplinary team.
- Disease-specific clinics may provide logistical problems in arranging a sufficient number of such clinics to cover the necessary range of disabilities and symptoms and thus there is a risk of ignoring the needs of people with rarer conditions.
- Some find it distressing to see individuals with the same condition in a more disabled state.
- Outpatient clinics are generally regarded as unsatisfactory by the users and many disability publications confirm this point.

Organizational models—primary care team

A typical group general practice in the UK has a population of around 10 000 people. The numbers of people requiring assistance from a rehabilitation team are reduced to a manageable number if the team is based within a typical general practice population. The *advantages* of the rehabilitation team being general practice-based are:

- The rest of the primary care team are on hand to deal with other general medical problems as and when they arise.
- People with disabilities tend not to be seen as a separate specific entity but are seen as part of the general population simply attending the GP's surgery as any other member of the public.
- The GP's surgery would tend to be local and usually reasonably accessible for the disabled person.
- The knowledge of the local primary care team should be increased by contact with local rehabilitation professionals.

However, there are some clear *disadvantages*:

- Many disabilities are quite rare. The GP, for example, is likely to only see one new person with multiple sclerosis every 20 years. Thus the level of expertise within the primary care team is strictly limited and undoubtedly the primary care team would need to be supplemented with appropriately trained rehabilitation staff.
- It is unlikely that necessary expertise and rehabilitation professionals could be provided for every primary care team. Recruitment and retention could be major problems.
- The local rehabilitation team could feel professionally isolated and slowly become deskilled if inadequate attention is paid to appropriate links with local and regional teams as well as specific time put aside for education and training.

However, there are many ways where a primary care team can be involved in the long-term management of people with physical disabilities. In one project, for example, a rehabilitation physician and a physiotherapist attend regular meetings with the primary care team to discuss management issues for people with Parkinson's disease. In another project the specialist rehabilitation team does outreach clinics in a GP's surgery. In a further project, in a large group general practice, one GP and one district nurse have been specifically trained by the regional rehabilitation team to manage the more routine and day-to-day difficulties encountered by disabled people—thus providing some local specialist knowledge to the local disabled population.

Organizational models—community rehabilitation team

In theory a full interdisciplinary rehabilitation team could be provided in the local community. The team would clearly need close liaison and good working relations with the local primary care team in that area as well as the local hospital unit and indeed the regional unit. Such an arrangement should overcome some of the disadvantages of the service being provided by the primary care team itself. One example, in Newcastle upon Tyne, is a local community multiple sclerosis team. The team has a physical base in the Rehabilitation Centre but assessment and ongoing therapy is mainly conducted in the individual's home. A weekly social/support group is run at the centre. The team itself, consisting of a physiotherapist (team manager), occupational therapist, therapy assistant, and secretary, are all employed on a full-time basis as well as part-time input from a counsellor, social worker, multiple sclerosis nurse, clinical neuropsychologist, and rehabilitation physician. The team has access to wider specialist support and respite beds are provided in a local rehabilitation centre. The team accepts referrals from a variety of sources, particularly GPs and neurologists as well as the local multiple sclerosis society (which part funds the team). The team has good links with local social services department and the necessity for double assessment by the health team and then the social services team is avoided. The potential disadvantages of such a team are:

- The team may have a health focus and thus less emphasis on important social and vocational issues.
- The team may only deal with a particular disability (such as multiple sclerosis) to the detriment of people with other diagnostic conditions.
- The provision of a comprehensive community rehabilitation team in every locality is unrealistic as sufficient numbers of trained staff would simply not be available—nor would there be the resources to pay for their services.

Organizational models—specialist therapists and nurses

If a full community rehabilitation team is unlikely to be provided in every locality then a somewhat less expensive possibility is to provide specially trained individual practitioners. In recent years there has been a growth of the concept of the specialist practitioner, particularly in a nursing context. There are now specially trained nurses with expertise in such conditions as Parkinson's disease, epilepsy, and multiple sclerosis as well as symptom-based specialist nurses working in the fields of, for example, continence and stoma care. There is now the emerging concept of a similar specialist therapist—such as physiotherapists with a particular expertise in the management of spasticity. While some of these specialist therapists and nurses are still hospital based many are now beginning to work in a community setting. Some are attached to the primary care team whilst others perform outreach work from the local, or the regional, rehabilitation centres. There are a number of *advantages* to this model:

- A broad range of disorders and symptoms can be covered.
- It is clearly less expensive to provide a single broadly trained practitioner in the community rather than the full community rehabilitation team.
- The practitioner can act as a contact point for people within their expert area. Many problems should be able to be dealt with by the practitioner, but onward referral to the local or regional teams could still be made.
- Close links can be maintained with the primary care team.
- Disabled people can be seen in their own home—thus saving unnecessary trips to hospital outpatient departments or unnecessary hospital admission.

However, there are obvious *disadvantages*:

- One individual cannot provide all the necessary expertise to an entire diagnostic group.
- Individuals are working in isolation and do not have the advantages of working as a member of an interdisciplinary rehabilitation team.
- Individuals would require lengthy training and considerable effort would need to be expended on continuing professional development. At the moment, at the least in the UK, such comprehensive training and support programmes are not yet widely available.

Given relatively limited resources in health, however, the concept of the independent specialist practitioner working in the community that links to the local and regional centre is a model worth pursuing as long as such development goes hand in hand with a proper high-quality training programme.

Organizational models—the Independent Living Movement and resource centres

There are now many examples of local authorities giving disabled people their own budget to buy in their own services. This is a model firmly supported by *the Independent Living Movement* and by disabled groups in general. A disabled individual will access their own appropriate parts of the community rehabilitation team and buy in their care within their own home. This is certainly a workable solution for many disabled people. However, problems do arise in some circumstances. People with cognitive or behavioural problems may have difficulty identifying their own requirements. This can raise difficult questions—who should manage their affairs and who should judge whether a given individual is able to manage their own budget or not? If an advocate is needed then such an advocate will need appropriate training so they know which services are on offer and which are appropriate. How does the system deal with inappropriate or unprovidable purchasing requests? What happens if there insufficient funds or an individual's budget becomes overspent? There are solutions to all these questions, and indeed this model can work quite well for many people. However, for everyone to buy in all the services they require will clearly need a very significant increase in available resources for the disabled population and difficulties with rationing would soon come into play.

If some facilities could be shared then this may alleviate some problems. One solution is to provide a *local community resource centre*. Such centres would be local, accessible, and house a range of facilities, including an information service and a disabled living centre, and would probably act as a base for local voluntary and self-help groups as well as a physical site for the local rehabilitation team. Outpatient clinics could be held in the centre from the local hospital or indeed outreach clinics from the regional centre. Social and recreational activities could be provided and other agencies could have an office in the centre, such as housing, social security, and employment services. The centres could, and probably should, be managed by and for disabled people. A number of such resource centres have now been established in the UK and abroad.

Community rehabilitation in developing countries

Most of the examples in the preceding sections are applicable to health systems in the Western world, particularly in Europe, the USA, Australia, and Canada. However, most of the rest of the world has less than adequate rehabilitation resources and facilities. Many people in developing countries have no access at all to any rehabilitation facility. If they are able to get in to a hospital rehabilitation unit then more often than not there is no community support after discharge. Thus, other models have been developed to overcome these difficulties in the developing world. The World Health Organization developed the concept of *community-based rehabilitation* (CBR). The model is open to different interpretations but the general approach is for the local community to be the main supporter of its own disabled population. Local village workers are given some basic disability training—perhaps just lasting a few weeks. In many parts of the world one or more individuals in the local village are already involved in some aspect of basic health care or child birth. These people are given further training, generally supported by non-governmental organizations, and are provided with further background disability knowledge. At this basic level of training it has been shown that such people can deal with about 80% of the needs of a disabled population in their own village. The village workers may need support and ongoing training and supervision which is usually provided by a more trained individual who covers a number of local villages—perhaps visiting them on a regular basis to deal with more complex problems and make appropriate referrals to the local hospital or a regional centre.

The CBR model has been developed in many places to establish disabled groups in individual villages to provide economically viable employment for themselves. The groups, perhaps with some external support, are trained and provided with basic tools for such skills as woodworking, dressmaking, and bicycle repairing. These groups then contribute a small sum to a central pool so that a few members of the group needing medicine or external referral can be supported. Obviously such basic training and support of disabled people is far from ideal but nevertheless such systems have been shown to be viable, cheap, and offer sustainable solutions for many disabled people in terms of health care and employment. The concept also goes some way to reducing the stigma of disability; disabled people in many cultures are marginalized from their own communities. There is a great need for much more to be done on a global basis and very significant investment is required in developing countries for the establishment of an appropriate disability infrastructure. However, CBR is a start and in many parts of the world is still the only means of long-term support for disabled people.

Further reading

1. Department of Health (2005). *The National Service Framework for long term conditions.* Department of Health, London. Available at 🕙 www.dh.gov.uk
2. Department of Health (2007). *Specialised Services National Definition Set: 7 Complex specialised rehabilitation for brain injury and complex disability (adult).* Available at 🕙 www.dh.gov.uk

Chapter 5

Assessment of disability

Why is disability assessment necessary?

Rehabilitation is a very complex activity and is difficult to quantify. Outcome measurement lacks the specificity seen in the treatment of pathology, but the World Health Organization's International Classification of Functioning, Disability and Health (ICF) has brought new ways of thinking. Rather than measure the activity of a pathology or disease, the focus is on the change in activity and participation as a consequence of the rehabilitation process, i.e. what is the added value of the rehabilitation given to a patient over and above a spontaneous recovery or improvement following an acute single injury or illness? Rehabilitation may slow down the deterioration and improve quality of life in patients with progressive disability, for which the measures used for static or improving conditions will not be appropriate. There are essentially five categories of patients (Box 5.1).

> **Box 5.1 Potential courses of health conditions**
>
> 1. Patients with potential to make a spontaneous full return to pre-morbid levels of health
> 2. Steadily improving patients, but may not return to pre-morbid levels of health and function
> 3. Patients not improving greatly, but with potential to improve
> 4. Slowly deteriorating patients, whose deterioration will be delayed by treatment and rehabilitation
> 5. Steadily or rapidly deteriorating patients despite rehabilitation interventions

Rehabilitation is effective in all, but rehabilitation units have to design different programmes for each. Measurement is thus important at a patient level to note a change in functioning, as well as at a health policy service level to assist in allocating funding for services. The ICF allows rehabilitation issues to be assessed for changes in impairments and functioning within the contextual factors for any patient or population of people at risk.

Measurement

Definitions

- Measurement—the use of a standard to quantify an observation.
- Measurement tools—the techniques used to quantify that observation.
- Outcome—the result obtained in using such instruments.

The essential measure in rehabilitation is to define the goals of rehabilitation for a particular patient and to determine whether or not the patient achieved the goals at the end of the rehabilitation episode. This is a measure of success, but the true value depends on the skill of the team in defining realistic, achievable, and desirable targets. If a goal is too easy, then the measure will have a ceiling effect, i.e. too many people will achieve the goal or the top of the scale, whereas if it is too difficult, the patient's actual achievements will not be amply recognized. Wade has detailed a number of measures in his book[1], but the most important factor is to measure something to show that the patient has changed because of the rehabilitation intervention and not despite it through natural recovery. One must therefore measure something that reflects the rehabilitation process and a number of items that show a change in ICF domains, i.e. in the patient's impairment and activity, in their participation and/or quality of life. Linear quantitative measures are *nominal, ordinal, interval, ratio and hierarchical* (Table 5.1).

The difficulty is how does the measurement of the sum of the individual components of an individually established rehabilitation programme reflect the client's goals? How does one separate out the impact of nursing or therapist interventions and, more importantly, how does one demonstrate its value (in terms of costs and quality) and its cost-effectiveness? The ideal scale should be sensitive, specific, reliable, appropriate, acceptable and robust. Each must be validated against standard criteria to which the attribute may be assessed. In disability research, false positive and false negative findings are common and a true positive rate (the sensitivity) needs to be compared against the false positive rate (i.e. the specificity). Not only must scores be valid, they must be reliable and consistent. They must also be reliable between raters as well as repeatable, so inter-rater reliability and test–retest reliability are of importance.

This chapter will look at some of these, but it is not a comprehensive list.

see Table 5.2, 5.3, 5.4.

Table 5.1 Linear quantitative measures of rehabilitation

Nominal scale	Classifies a characteristic number along a straight line. Points on the scale have no meaning within the context in which they are being used, but may be useful if the frequencies of that particular characteristic are being studied.
Ordinal scale	Ranks the order, so that each adjacent score measures a parameter along a line, i.e. one point above or below is higher or lower than the last e.g. the Visual Analogue Scale, the Barthel Index, and the Functional Independence Measurement (FIM).
Interval scale	Common interval—constant unit of measurement between one point and another—with arbitrary zero point, as perhaps are the units of measurement.
Ratio scale	Interval scale with a true zero at its origin, e.g. measuring weight, cost per case.
Hierarchical scale	Natural hierarchy, e.g. each point on rising scale indicates a greater ability or skill than the last.

Goal Attainment Scale (GAS)

First introduced by Kirusek colleagues[2] for assessing outcomes for complex interventions in mental health settings, it has now been used in many other areas of rehabilitation. It scores the extent to which patient's individual goals are achieved in the course of an intervention. Tasks are individually identified to suit the patient, and the levels are individually set around their current and expected levels of performance. It focuses on outcomes important to the patient and relevant to the treatment. The patient is actively involved in determining the goals and evaluating their achievement. As it depends on the multidisciplinary team's (MDT's) ability to predict outcomes, it should be supported by other standardized outcome measures. Each goal is rated on a 5-point scale, with the degree of attainment captured for each goal area (Box 5.2):

Box 5.2 5-point GAS score

Score	Goal
−2	Current status and abilities
−1	Improved but has not achieved goal set
0	Specific goal achieved
+1	Somewhat better
+2	Much better

Goals may be weighted to take account of the relative importance of the goal to the individual, and/or the anticipated difficulty of achieving it. The overall GASs are then calculated by applying a formula[3]:

$$\text{Overall GAS} = 50 + \frac{10\Sigma \, (w_i \underline{x}_i)\ldots\ldots}{[(1-\rho) \, \Sigma \, w_i{}^2 + \rho(\Sigma \, (w_i)^2)]^{\frac{1}{2}}}$$

(w_i = the weight assigned to the ith goal (if equal weights, w_i = 1); $\underline{x}_i$ = the numerical value achieved (between −2 and +2); ρ = the expected correlation of the goal scales.

Table 5.2 Scales used to measure different disability domains

Domain	Impairment	Function and participation
Mobility	Power, e.g. MRC Scale (see Box 5.3) Spasticity—Ashworth (see Box 5.4) and Tardieu Scales, Wartenburg Test Motricity Index—lower and upper limb	Walking speed and distance time 'Time to get up and go' test
Upper limb and hand	Grip strength—dynamometry, crude, but simple to perform; using a small cuff and sphygmomanometer is useful in clinical practice.	Nine-hole peg test Assesses the ability to perform coordinated fine movements Measures the time taken to place nine pegs in nine holes Test should be terminated if it is not completed in 50 seconds.
Function	Physiological cost index (PCI) = activity pulse rate − rest rate / speed of activity	
Communication	Frenchay Aphasia Screening Test (FAST) Boston Aphasia Screening Test	
Cognition	Mini-Mental State Examination Hodkinson Mental Test Score	Digit span—a test of attention within the Weschler Adult Intelligence Scale (WAIS)
Mood	Hospital Anxiety and Depression Test	
Disability	Activities of daily living	OPCS Disability Scale Barthel Score Functional Independence Measure (FIM) Nottingham Extended ADL Scale London Handicap Scale Sickness Impact Scale

Box 5.3 MRC Scale
0 No muscular activity
1 Minimal contraction of muscle but insufficient to move a joint
2 Contraction of muscle sufficient to move a joint but not oppose gravity
3 Muscle contraction sufficient to move a joint against gravity but not against physical resistance
4 Muscle contraction sufficient to move a joint against gravity and against mild/moderate resistance
4+ Muscle contraction sufficient to move a joint against gravity and against greater resistance than in level 4
5 Normal power, i.e. muscular contraction sufficient to resist firm resistance

Box 5.4 Modified Ashworth Scale
(adapted from Bohannon and Smith (1986)[4])
4 Rigid extremity
3 Loss of full joint movement, difficult movement, considerable tone.
2 Full joint/limb movement, but more marked increase in tone, limb still easily moved
1+ Slight increase in tone, catch and resistance throughout range of movement.
1 Slight increase in tone, catch, or minimal resistance at end of range of movement.
0 No increase in tone

References

1. Wade DT (1992). *Measurement in Neurological Rehabilitation*. Oxford University Press, Oxford.
2. Lombillo JR, Kirusek TJ, and Sherman RE (1973). Evaluation a community mental health program, contract fulfilment analysis. Hospital and community psychiatry **24** (11), 760–762.
3. Turner-Stokes L et al. (in press). *The Management of Adults With Spasticity Using Botulinum Toxin: A Guide To Clinical Practice.*
4. Bohannon RW and Smith MB (1986). Interrater reliability of a modified Ashworth scale of muscle spasticity. *Physical Therapy*, **67**, 206–7.

Examples

Communication

Dysphasia can be screened using the Frenchay Aphasia Screening Test (FAST). This is the ability to record a set of pictures and is clinically a useful bedside test. It correlates with the Boston Aphasia Screening Test, which is regularly used by speech and language therapists.

Cognitive measures

The Mini-Mental State Examination is widely used as screening test of cognitive impairment. It includes an assessment of many elements of higher cerebral functions, such as memory, attention, and language. It is a useful basic tool for inclusion in a battery of tests of cognitive function. However, the Hodkinson Mental Test and the digit span, which is a test of attention within the Weschler Adult Intelligence Scale (WAIS), are valuable at the bedside.

Hodkinson score

The patient scores 1 for correct answers to the following questions:-
- Age of patient.
- Time (to nearest hour).
- An address given for recall at end of test.
- Name of hospital/area of town.
- Year.
- Month.
- Patient's date of birth.
- Dates of significant event, e.g. World War II.
- Name of monarch/prime minister.
- Count backwards from 20 to 1 (no errors but may correct self).

The Hospital Anxiety and Depression Scale is useful in stroke rehabilitation, but its value diminishes thereafter. A score of 7 or below for anxiety/depression is normal, though scores of 11 or above are abnormal.

Activities of daily living (ADL)

The Modified Barthel Index (Table 5.3) has been validated in stroke patients and is predictive at 1 month for functional independence at 6 months. It, however, does not take into account difficulties with communication, cognition, and mood, but is simple, reliable, and quick to carry out. It should measure what the patient 'does do' rather than what he or she 'can do' and thus an element of hierarchical significance appears. The maximum score is 20.

The Functional Independence Measure (FIM) consists of 18 subsets measured on a scale of 1 to 7 (1 being total care required, to 7 being full independence). The Functional Assessment Measure (FAM) has been added to the FIM to accommodate the burden of care in traumatic brain injury. This uses the same criteria but the FAM measures extend activities of daily living to cover community mobility and cognitive features which are relevant to post-acute traumatic brain injury rehabilitation. The FIM + FAM is only validated for inpatient settings and is designed to be performed by the whole rehabilitation team. It is also designed to give information for the planning of rehabilitation goals and scores can be displayed in such a way that deficits can be easily identified. Rehabilitation units in the UK are gaining experience with this measure and it has become one of a basket of measures undertaken.

Participation

Several scales have been derived from the original WHO ICIDH text referring to orientation, physical independence, mobility, occupation, social integration, and economic self-sufficiency, of which the London Handicap Scale and the Edinburgh Rehabilitation Status Scale have become best known. The Frenchay Activities Index measures social integration (a measure of a person's behaviour and therefore, in the absence of mental illness or a personality disorder, a useful measure of social function). Well-being is difficult to measure in either health or social settings and many profiles have been devised to identify subjective views on how well people feel and how satisfied they are with life. The Sickness Impact Profile and the SF36 are examples and the latter has been used widely in patients with musculoskeletal problems.

Rasch analysis

This is a method of taking disparate values and organizing them in to a measurement tool that makes sense. It is useful in rehabilitation as it can cover individual items and give some weighting in order to identify charac-teristics to guide the rehabilitation process.

Table 5.3 Modified Barthel Index

Bowels	Bladder
0 = Incontinent (or needs enemas)	0 = Incontinent/ catheterized
1 = Occasional accident (once a week)	1 = Occasional accident (max. once/ 24 hours)
2 = Continent	2 = Continent

Grooming	Toilet use
0 = Needs help with personal care	0 = Dependent
1 = Independent face/hair/teeth/ shaving	1 = Needs help but can do something alone
	2 = Independent (on and off, dressing, wiping)

Feeding	Transfer
0 = Unable	0 = Unable, no sitting balance
1 = Needs help with cutting, spreading etc.	1 = Major help from 1 or 2 people, can sit
2 = Independent	2 = Minor help (verbal or physical)
	3 = Independent

Mobility	Stairs
0 = Immobile	0 = Unable
1 = Wheelchair independent, including corners	1 = Needs help (verbal, physical)
2 = Walks with help of 1 person (verbal/physical)	2 = Independent
3 = Independent but may use any aid	

Dressing	Bathing
0 = Dependent	0 = Dependent
1 = Needs help but can do half unaided	1 = Independent or in shower
2 = Independent including buttons, zips, laces etc.	

Table 5.4 Nottingham Extended ADL Index

Questions—Do you...? (scoring)	Not at all 1	With help 2	Alone with difficulty 3	Alone easily 4
Mobility				
Walk around outside?				
Climb stairs?				
Get in and out of the car?				
Walk over uneven ground?				
Cross roads?				
Travel on public transport?				
Kitchen				
Manage to feed yourself?				
Manage to make yourself a hot drink?				
Take hot drinks from one room to another?				
Do the washing up?				
Make yourself a hot snack?				
Domestic tasks				
Manage your own money when you are out?				
Wash small items of clothing?				
Do a full clothes wash?				
Leisure activity				
Read newspapers or books?				
Use the telephone?				
Write letters?				
Go out socially?				
Manager your own garden?				
Drive a car?				

Further reading

1. Wade DT (1992). *Measurement in Neurological Rehabilitation.* Oxford University Press, Oxford.

Chapter 6

Spasticity

Definition

Spasticity is one of the most commonly encountered problems in the field of neurological rehabilitation. It is a significant factor that can reduce functional mobility and is a major impediment in the rehabilitation process. Untreated or badly treated spasticity can lead to joint contractures which in turn cause problems in maintaining a suitable posture for feeding, communication, and many aspects of daily living. Muscle spasms, often associated with spasticity, can be painful and one of the predisposing causes for the development of pressure sores. The proper treatment of spasticity is not difficult and can be very beneficial for the overall quality of life. It is one of the more rewarding challenges for the rehabilitation team.

What is spasticity?

It has been defined[1] as *a motor disorder characterized by a velocity-dependent increase in tonic stretch reflexes with exaggerated tendon jerks*. However, this rather bland definition hides the fact that spasticity occurs in a bewildering variety of different forms. It is usually accompanied by various other features of the upper motor neuron (UMN) syndrome (□ see p.88). A new definition of spasticity was tabled by Pandyan *et al.* in 2005[2] to describe the entire range of signs and symptoms that are collectively described as the positive features of the upper motor neuron (UMN) syndrome but narrows the term to exclude the negative features and the pure biomechanical changes in soft tissues and joints.

Features of spasticity

Spasticity is nearly always accompanied by impairment of voluntary muscle activation. Such impairment will vary, but can include weakness, slowness in building up to maximal power, and clumsiness of voluntary movements. This clumsiness usually results from impaired coordination of the synergistic agonist muscles as well as involving inappropriate restraint or failure of inhibition of the muscles whose action antagonizes the intended movement. The range of voluntary movement that can be achieved is sometimes reduced to just a small number of stereotyped patterns—the so-called *spastic synergies*.

Presentation

Spasticity is usually demonstrated by imposing a passive movement on a limb and thus inducing involuntary activation of the stretched muscle. Response is usually *velocity dependent* being larger in response to a rapid stretch than a slow stretch. The stretch may trigger a '*spasm*' which is an involuntary and usually self-limiting co-activation of agonist and antagonist muscles of one or more limbs, which can sometimes involve girdle or trunk muscles that are anatomically close to the limbs affected. These spasms are sometimes triggered by cutaneous stimulation. In extensor muscles, especially in the legs, a characteristic pattern is often known as the '*clasp knife response*'. When the muscle is stretched progressively from its shortened position its initial response is the usual velocity-sensitive resistance. However, once a certain length is achieved all resistance dies away and the extensor muscle becomes flaccid only to resume this activation when allowed to shorten. If these features are put together with the other positive and negative features present in the

UMN syndrome then it can be seen that spasticity can cause a bewildering variety of different clinical problems.

Neurophysiology

At a basic neurophysiological level it has been shown that the alpha motor neurons serving skeletal muscle are hyperexcitable in spasticity and are thus activated by inputs that would not normally provoke any response. In many cases this hyperexcitability is facilitated by the lack of descending inhibitory input from the cortex or higher in the spinal cord. Measures that reduce the activity of the reflex loop from 1a afferent nerve fibres through to the alpha motor neurons can be effective in reducing spasticity. Thus, agents which block sensory inputs such as local anaesthetics or neurolytic drugs, or those which potentiate presynaptic inhibition such as baclofen, have all been shown to reduce the intensity of muscle activation in response to passive stretch. This is a rather simplistic view of neurophysiology of spasticity but nevertheless the over-activity of the afferent/ efferent reflex arc at the spinal level provides a model upon which some logical treatment can be based.

Hypertonia and spasticity

- It is important to clarify the difference between increased tone or hypertonia, and spasticity. These terms are often used interchangeably leading to confusion regarding the patient's presenting symptoms and subsequent appropriate treatment.
- Hypertonia can be defined as the sensation of resistance that is encountered as a joint is passively moved through a range of motion. Thus the velocity is unimportant. It can be contributed to the biomechanical changes that occur in muscle, soft tissues and joint following immobilization.
- Hypertonia can be caused by a combination of neural (spasticity) and non-neural components.

References

1. Lance JW (1980). Symposium synopsis in: Feloman RG, Young RR, voella WP (eds). *Spasticity disorder of motor control*. Year book medical publishers: Chicago pp. 485–494.
2. Pandyan AD, Gregoric M, Barnes MP, et al. (2005). Spasticity: Clinical perceptions, neurological realities and meaningful measurement. *Disability and Rehabilitation*, **27**, 2–6.

Upper motor neuron syndrome

Spasticity is just one of various phenomena that are associated with a UMN lesion. The UMN syndrome is a collection of problems that can occur with any lesion or disturbance of the UMN pathway. UMN lesions cause a variety of both positive and negative features (Table 6.1).

Thus there is a wide range of disturbances in the UMN syndrome and only one such disturbance is spasticity. In general terms there are many treatment possibilities for the positive features of the UMN syndrome but there are limitations in terms of treatment for the negative features. When treating spasticity the other features of the UMN syndrome that may or may not be present in the individual can have a profound influence on the response to treatment.

Table 6.1 Positive and negative features of UMN lesions

Negative features	Muscle weakness
	Loss of dexterity
	Fatigability
Positive features	Increased tendon reflexes with radiation
	Clonus
	Positive Babinsky sign
	Spasticity
	Extensor spasms
	Flexor spasms
	Mass reflex
	Dyssynergic patterns of co-contraction during movement
	Associated reactions and other dyssynergic and stereotypical spastic patterns

Further reading

1. Barnes MP, Johnson GR (ed.) (2008). *Upper motor neurone syndrome and spasticity. Clinical management and neurophysiology*, 2nd edn. Cambridge University Press, Cambridge.

Goals of treatment and outcome measures

The treatment of spasticity, like all rehabilitation processes, should start with the establishment of specific achievable goals and a carefully planned strategy to achieve those goals.

First, does the spasticity need treating at all? Although spasticity is an abnormal neurophysiological event it can still be a positive phenomenon for a given individual. Spasticity in the leg, for example, may serve as a brace to support weight whilst walking or transferring. Arm spasticity can sometimes be useful for assisting in dressing. Some treatments of spasticity can also produce significant side effects. The oral anti-spastic agents, for example, can induce weakness and fatigue which overall can be more detrimental than leaving the spasticity untreated. In general the goals of treatment of spasticity can be:

• To enable carrying out of personal-care tasks and dressing.
• To maintain skin integrity.
• To improve function.
• To reduce the risk of unnecessary complications.
• To alleviate pain.

Sometimes a goal of the treatment of spasticity is not actually to assist the person with spasticity. Sometimes spasticity can make nursing care particularly difficult. Every time the person is moved a spasm can be induced which can make positioning in bed or a chair or on the toilet extraordinarily difficult. The person themselves may not be particularly bothered by the spasticity or may even be unaware of its presence. A valid reason for treatment is sometimes to ease nursing care in order to assist with the management of hygiene, dressing, and transferring.

Once the goal has been established then a suitable outcome measure needs to be chosen. There are a few documented reliable measures of spasticity but most are really only appropriate in a research setting. The commonest scale is the Ashworth Scale (📖 see Box 5.4, p.78). There are problems with this scale but nevertheless it is still the most widely used. However, in practical clinical terms it is sometimes valid to use a simple measure that is relevant to the functional goal. If, for example, the aim of treatment is to reduce pain then a simple visual analogue pain scale could be used as an outcome measure. If the aim is to improve walking then a simple 10-minute, timed walking test may suffice. The outcome measure should be simple and practical and obviously relevant to the stated aim of treatment and most importantly the patient and/or carer.

Finally it should be remembered that spasticity is a dynamic phenomenon. It can vary not only according to posture but also according to degree of fatigue, timing of medication, and even the weather. Thus, assessment sometimes needs to be a rather prolonged process with observation of the individual at different times of the day. A quick bedside or outpatient clinic examination is often insufficient and can lead to inappropriate treatment.

This, however, does not differentiate between the resistance from neural or biomechanical contributions. The Tardieu Scale appears to be better at identifying the neural component but is still not in wide use (📖 see The Tardieu Scale, p.92).

Further reading

1. Morris S (2002). Ashworth and Tardieu Scales: Their clinical relevance for measuring spasticity in adult and paediatric neurological populations. *Physical Therapy Reviews*, **7**, 53–62.

The Tardieu Scale

Criteria for performing the Tardieu Scale

Grading is always performed at the same time of day, in a constant position of the body for a given limb. Other joints, particularly the neck, must also remain in a constant position throughout the test and between tests. For each muscle group, reaction to stretch is rated at a specified stretch to velocity with two parameters X and Y.

- The patient is positioned in sitting for upper limbs.
- Lower limbs are tested in supine.

Criteria for scoring the Tardieu Scale

Velocity to stretch:

- V1: as slow as possible.
- V2: speed of the limb segment falling under gravity.
- V3: as fast as possible (faster than the rate of the natural drop of the limb segment under gravity).
- V1 is used to measure the passive range of motion (PROM).
- Only V2 and V3 are used to rate spasticity.

Quality of muscle reaction (X)

- 0: no resistance throughout the course of the passive movement.
- 1: slight resistance throughout the course of the passive movement, with no clear catch at precise angle.
- 2: clear catch at precise angle, interrupting the passive movement, followed by release.
- 3: fatigable clonus (<10 seconds when maintaining pressure) occurring at precise angle.
- 4: infatigable clonus (>10 seconds when maintaining pressure) occurring at precise angle.

Angle of muscle reaction (Y)

Measured relative to the position of minimal stretch of the muscle (corresponding to angle) where it is relative to the resting anatomic position.

References

1. Tardieu G, Shentoub S, Delarue R (1954). Alarecherched'une technique de mesure de la spasticite Rev Neurol **91**, 143–144.

Further reading

1. Morris S (2002). Ashworth and Tardieu Scales: Their clinical relevance for measuring spasticity in adult and paediatric neurological populations. *Physical Therapy Reviews*, **7**, 53–62.
2. Stevenson VL, Jarrett L (ed.) (2006). *Spasticity management. A practical multidisciplinary guide.* Informa Healthcare.
3. ⌂ www.mdvu.org/library/disease/spasticity—a useful online resource library.
4. ⌂ www.wemove.org—an excellent website providing information for patient care and health care professionals.

Treatment strategies—alleviation of exacerbating factors and positioning

Alleviation of exacerbating factors

There are many external stimuli that can exacerbate and aggravate spasticity. Common causes include:

- Distension or infection of the bladder.
- Constipation.
- Skin irritations, such as in-growing toenails and pressure sores.
- Increased sensory stimuli from external causes, including ill-fitting orthotic appliances, catheter leg bags, and tight clothing or footwear.
- Inappropriate seating or bad positioning in a wheelchair.
- In people who are comatosed or cognitively disturbed then exacerbation of spasticity could be due to underlying abdominal emergency or lower limb fracture.

Sometimes attention to these details can be sufficient to treat the spasticity without other intervention.

Positioning

Probably the most important yet simple treatment is proper seating of the individual. The supine position that is so commonly adopted in the early stages after stroke or brain injury when the person is spending a long time in bed can simply exacerbate extensor spasm by facilitation of the *tonic labyrinthine supine reflex*. Simply sitting the person in a more upright position can avoid this posture and reduce spasticity. In other people, particularly in the early stages after brain injury, an *asymmetric tonic neck reflex* is present. This means if the head is turned to one side then the hip assumes a flexed position in abduction and external rotation whilst the other hip assumes an adducted and internally rotated posture. This is a common cause of later orthopaedic problems, especially in children where it can lead to subluxation of the hip on the adducted side. Awareness of this reflex can prevent the problem.

Treatment strategies—physiotherapy

The most valuable member of the rehabilitation team in terms of treatment of spasticity is the physiotherapist. The physiotherapist has a key role in the following areas:

- Initial assessment to determine the level of spasticity:
  - Muscle activity/weakness.
  - Muscle length/shortening.
  - Presence of pain.
  - Available function.

A treatment plan to address the problems identified can then be instigated which may include the following:

- Positioning programmes—can be instigated following initial baseline assessment to ascertain current position, current tonal and musculo-skeletal problems and then implement change. To be effective 24-hour management is essential by the team and there is now a wide selection of positioning equipment available to facilitate postural change, e.g. sleep systems, T-rolls, and wedge cushions.
- Seating—should be seen as a tool to apply a specific intended stimulus for a corrective purpose such as normalizing alignment and or reducing abnormal tone. Considerations when seating clients should be made to:
  - Importance of base of support/pelvic stabilization.
  - Importance of symmetry and head and neck alignment.
  - Inhibition of tonal patterns.
  - Range of movement.
  - Levels of fatigue and loss of activity.
  - An extensive range of wheelchairs are now available to assist with postural support and correction, e.g.
    – Tilt-in-space chairs.
    – Recliners.
    – Chairs with moulded inserts.
    – Powerchairs.
- Stretching programmes—are crucial to maintain and alter muscle length, however the evidence is still varied regarding the optimum length of time for a muscle to be stretched, ranging from 6 hours per day[1] to more recent evidence (in 2005) of 30 minutes per day[2]. Even at the minimum of 30 minutes for each muscle this is impossible to be carried out manually by a physiotherapist hence the use of tilt tabling, serial casting, splinting, and positional programmes.
- Serial casting—used to improve muscle length and joint range. Application of serial casts made of plaster of Paris or soft cast have been shown to increase the number of sarcomeres and reduce spasticity. They can be changed every 3–5 days over several weeks until the desired range is achieved. Serial casting is most commonly used for elbows, knees, and ankles.
- Physiotherapy approaches—there are many schools of physiotherapy which claim that a particular technique has anti-spastic and functional benefits. The Bobath technique is widely used, but there are other schools including proprioceptive neuromuscular facilitation and motor learning. There is very little evidence that any particular technique is more efficacious than another and many neurological physiotherapists

will now use an eclectic selection of different dynamic approaches to ease spasticity and improve functional gait for a given person.
• Functional electrical stimulation—shown to enhance the effect of botulinum and improve the reduction of spasticity in targeted muscles as well as being used to facilitate and strengthening the agonist when the antagonist muscle has been injected.
• Targeted strengthening programmes—once taboo in the neuro-physiotherapy world have proven to be effective in reducing disability as increasing evidence shows weakness to be the main contributor to activity limitations rather than spasticity.
• Constraint induced therapy in combination with botulinum toxin—has shown increased use and function in the upper limb of chronic stroke patients.
• Orthotics—used to maintain or improve joint range and alignment and facilitate function, e.g. ankle foot orthosis, aircast splints, hand splints.
• Advice and instruction on home exercise and stretching programmes.

References

1. Tardieu C, Lespargot A, Tabary C, Bret M.O et al. (1988). For how long must the soleus muscle be stretched each day to prevent contracture? *Developmental Medicine and Child Neurology*, **30**, 3–10.
2. Ada L, Goddard E, McCully J, Stavrinost T, Bampton J et al. (2005). Thirty minutes of positioning reduces the development of shoulder external rotation contraction after stroke: A randomized controlled trial. *Archives of Physical Medicine and Rehabilitation*, **86**, 230–4.

Treatment strategies—oral medication

Oral medication can bring considerable problems. All anti-spastic drugs can induce weakness and fatigability. Sometimes these side effects are more troublesome than the original spasticity and all drugs should be used with care and constantly monitored. Available drugs are:

* Diazepam— this was the first anti-spastic agent to be used and probably has an anti-spastic effect by enhancing the action of the inhibiting neurotransmitter gamma aminobutyric acid (GABA). It is certainly an anti-spastic agent but often induces unacceptable weakness and tiredness and is now rarely used. Starting dose 2mg twice daily and then slowly increased by 2mg increments up to a maximum dose of 40–60mg per day in divided doses.

* Baclofen—this is probably the most widely used oral anti-spastic drug. It is a GABA B receptor agonist that may also work by a presynaptic inhibitory effect on the release of excitatory neurotransmitters such as a glutamate, aspartate, and substance P. It has a number of side effects common to most anti-spastic drugs, including drowsiness, fatigue, and muscle weakness. All these side effects are dose dependent and unfortunately there is only a narrow therapeutic window between benefit and unacceptable side effects. Most people need between 40 and 80mg of baclofen daily in divided doses. The drug should be introduced slowly and withdrawn equally slowly.

* Dantrolene sodium—this is a less useful anti-spastic medication. However, the mode of action is peripheral and it has a direct effect on skeletal muscle. Thus, there is a possibility of having a synergistic effect with other centrally acting agents. It has the usual range of side effects but in addition can cause hepatoxicity and liver function needs monitoring at regular intervals. Side effects are reduced if the drug is slowly increased, starting at 25mg daily and increased over several weeks to a maximum of around 400mg daily in divided doses.

Newer oral anti-spastic drugs

Tizanidine has fairly recently been introduced into the USA and UK although it has been available in some countries for a number of years. The mode of action is largely unknown, but it probably impairs excitatory amino acid release from spinal interneurons, amongst other actions. It seems to be similarly efficacious to baclofen but induces less weakness and is reasonably well tolerated. However, it still has a number of side effects including dry mouth, fatigue, and dizziness and, like dantrolene sodium, it can be associated with hepatoxicity and liver function needs regular monitoring.

The most effective dose should be determined for each patient and a titration period of 2–4 weeks appears adequate to ascertain optimal therapeutic dosage. It is usually initiated at 2mg twice daily and increased in 4mg increments every 4 to 7 days to a maximum of 36mg per day, divided into 3 or 4 doses.

Other anti-spastic drugs

There is a whole range of other anti-spastic agents that have been the subject of studies in the literature. However, few have stood the test of time. The agents that are still available and might be useful include:

- Cannabis—cannabis is likely to be an approved drug in the UK by 2009. There is evidence that it has useful anti-spastic properties as well as being anti-emetic and analgesic. It may turn out to be a useful anti-spastic medication once larger studies have been conducted.
- Clonidine.
- Levodopa.
- Gabapentin—this drug, originally marketed as an anti-convulsant, is showing promising results as an anti-spastic agent as well as being a neuralgic analgesic. It is generally well tolerated and is a useful addition to our armoury of oral anti-spastic agents.
  - Dosage – starting at 300mg increasing slowly by 300mg increments up to a maximum dose of 3600mg. Spasticity often lessened between 1800mg and 2400mg.
  - Side effects—drowsiness and balance disturbance.
- Pregabalin is an alternative to gabapentin.

Focal treatment—phenol and botulinum toxin

Most spasticity is focal and just affects one or a few muscle groups. The obvious problem with oral therapy is that it has a generalized systemic effect whereas the aim of treatment is to have an anti-spastic effect only on the spastic muscles. Thus, focal techniques have been developed which avoid the necessity for oral systemic drugs.

Phenol or alcohol nerve blocks

This simple technique involves blockage of a peripheral nerve by injection of phenol or alcohol. Any peripheral nerve that is readily accessible by needle can be blocked. The most useful nerves are:

• Obturator nerve—for adductor spasticity.
• Posterior tibial nerve—for calf spasticity.
• Sciatic nerve—for hamstring spasticity.
• Median, ulnar, or musculocutaneous nerves—for flexor arm spasticity.

The technique is simple and involves injection of the chemical through a needle electrode. The tip of the needle is manipulated to as close as possible to the nerve and its position is confirmed by electrical stimulation. A small volume of phenol or alcohol is then injected down the same needle. This produces an immediate nerve block with relaxation of the supplied muscle. The block will usually last 2–3 months but is sometimes permanent. The technique can be time-consuming and is sometimes uncomfortable. There can be problems with the effect of the block as sometimes a short-term block is needed in recoverable conditions and in such circumstances a long-term block needs to be avoided—but cannot be guaranteed. If a mixed motor/sensory nerve is injected then there can be troublesome sensory side effects including painful dysaesthesiae which can be permanent. However, the overriding advantage is that the technique is simple and cheap and thus can be used in health systems with limited resources.

Botulinum toxin*

Botulinum toxin is a potent neurotoxin that blocks the release of acetyl choline from nerve endings. The toxin is available in fixed-dose ampoules and will normally require reconstitution in normal saline. The reconstituted solution is then injected directly into the spastic muscle. The toxin will spread within the muscle and over the course of 2–3 days will induce a local relaxation. This anti-spastic effect lasts around 2–3 months before the injection needs repeating. The technique is quick, simple, and effective and there are usually no side effects. A small number of people can develop a flu-like illness. The main problem is over-relaxation of the muscle inducing unnecessary weakness but with a careful technique this is unusual. However, the toxin is very expensive and is not likely to be used in countries where resources are scarce.

In the long term about 5–10% of people on repeat botulinum toxin injections develop clinical resistance. This is likely to be due to the development of antibodies to the toxin. The most commonly used toxin is type-A toxin (Dysport® or Botox®). Botulinum toxin type B (NeuroBloc® or Myobloc®)

is now available which in some people can overcome the problem of resistance. However, the type-B toxin does not seem as effective as the type-A toxin and there are a number of troublesome side effects, including severe dry mouth and pain on injection.

Despite these difficulties botulinum toxin has revolutionized the treatment of spasticity and in many people is now the treatment of choice, after simple measures and physiotherapy, for the management of focal spasticity.

*Readers should consult manufacturer's literature for a current range of licensed indications of each product.

Intrathecal techniques

Intrathecal baclofen

Another way of getting around the problem of oral medication is to inject an anti-spastic agent directly on to the spinal cord. The use of intrathecal baclofen was first described in 1984[1]. This technique involves:

• The implantation of a subcutaneous pump.
• A silastic catheter leading from the pump into the intrathecal space.

The pump is fully programmable and allows the constant infusion of a small dose of baclofen on to the spinal cord. The technique can be useful, particularly in severe and resistant spasticity. It is particularly useful for lower limb spasticity, but intrathecal baclofen will also affect the upper limbs. However, there are disadvantages:

• A surgical procedure is required.
• There is a risk of catheter movement.
• There is a risk of pump failure leading to no dosage or over-dosage of baclofen.
• The reservoir will need replenishing.

Intrathecal phenol

In some people with very severe spasticity with no motor, sensory, bowel, or bladder function intrathecal phenol can be injected into the lumbar spine to destroy the peripheral nerves and the cauda equina. This works very well in people who are already paraplegic and incontinent but obviously is reserved for people with the most severe problems of spasticity. There is some risk of pressure sores as all sensation below the injected level will be removed.

References

1. Penn RD, Kroin JS (1984). Intrathecal Baclofen alleviates spinal cord spasticity. *Lancet*, 8385–1078.

Surgical and orthopaedic procedures

If spasticity is treated properly in the first instance then it is unusual for a person to require surgery. However, surgery is sometimes required in people with severe or resistant spasticity. It is also required for the management of existing contractures. There are a number of anti-spastic surgical procedures:

- Anterior and posterior rhizotomy—involves section of the spinal reflex arc by cutting the relevant nerves.
- Microsurgical lesions of the dorsal route entry zone (drezotomy)—this is a slightly less invasive technique.
- Percutaneous radiofrequency rhizotomy—an even less invasive technique. It also disrupts the spinal reflex arc.
- Spinal cord and cerebellar stimulation—this is effective but does involve considerable problems with regard to surgery, equipment failure, and expense.

Sometimes surgical repositioning of joints and limbs is necessary for severe spasticity in order to facilitate proper seating, to ease positioning, to apply orthoses, and reduce the likelihood of further complications. There various orthopaedic interventions but the commonest are:

- Achilles tendon lengthening—for fixed equinus and equinovarus deformities.
- Adductor tenotomies or obturator neurectomies—for severe adductor spasticity.
- Cutting of hamstring tendons or hamstring lengthening procedures—for flexion deformities of the knees.

Upper limb surgery

Surgery in the arm is much more difficult and less successful than in the lower limb, but various tenotomy and tendon lengthening procedures are possible including:

- Lengthening of the biceps and brachioradialis—for elbow flexion deformity.
- Lengthening of the flexor carpi ulnaris and flexor carpi radialis—for wrist flexor spasticity.
- Transfer of the flexor pollicis longus to the radial side of the thumb—for isolated thumb-in-palm deformities.

Shoulder surgery is even more difficult but there are procedures including tenotomy of the pectoralis major, subscapularis, and lattisimus dorsi for severe internal rotation of the shoulder.

This is not a definitive review of surgical techniques for the management of spasticity but gives some idea of potential surgical interventions. However, it is important to emphasize that proper treatment in the early stages of spasticity should mean that surgery is rarely needed.

Chapter 7

Continence

Introduction

Neural control of the bladder and bowel extends from the frontal lobes to the sacral cord. Incontinence results from failure of control and is a major disabling problem. Bladder dysfunction is extremely common in many neurological diseases and following trauma. It is one of the most distressing impairments, which can give rise to considerable disability. Treatment may be complex, but it can often be greatly assisted by fairly simple means. Two major goals exist in clinical settings:

- Management of symptoms, particularly the incontinence itself.
- Minimization of kidney damage.

Renal failure has been a major cause of mortality in neurologically impaired patients, e.g. after spinal cord injury, and proper attention through rehabilitation, urological assessment, and follow-up can prevent this, so that renal compromise and death are rare (Box 7.1). If they do occur, it nowadays reflects inadequate care. Faecal incontinence is managed for its devastating impact on socialization rather than its risk to health.

> **Box 7.1 Prevalence in neurologically disabled people and in the elderly with multi-organ failure:**
> - Urinary—generally unknown, but common.
> - Faecal—considerably less common—feature of autonomic failure, e.g. in diabetes mellitus.

Normal bladder function

The anatomy and physiology are complex (Fig. 7.1). The bladder is composed of detrusor muscle, which allows urine to be collected and the bladder to expand without a rise in pressure until voiding is imminent. The bladder smooth muscle contracts to start voiding and the striated fibres of the external sphincter, which is separately innervated, relax.

Neural innervation

Autonomic nerve supply

The main nerve supply to the body of the detrusor muscles is from parasympathetic neurons lying in the cord at S2/3/4 level. The bladder, particularly the neck, also receives a supply from the thoraco lumbar sympathetic chain. The post-ganglionic sympathetic fibres are *adrenergic*, whereas the pre-ganglionic sympathetic fibres and parasympathetic fibres are *cholinergic*. Other neurotransmitters are involved, but this simple classification is useful when considering treatment

Somatic nerves

The urethral sphincter has a motor innervation from the discrete Onuf's nucleus at the S2/3/4 level in the cord. This is integrated with the parasympathetic supply, which also arises in this vicinity, and the motor fibres pass into the pudendal nerve, which supplies both the urethral and anal sphincters.

Sensory nerves

Bladder sensation is mostly conveyed via the pelvic and pudendal nerves to the spinal cord and upwards via the lateral spinothalamic tract. Afferent fibres will synapse in Onuf's nucleus to form a simple spinal reflex as well as also synapsing with the sympathetic chain.

Pontine micturition centre

This provides a coordinating function regulating long spinal reflexes and receiving modulatory (mainly inhibitory) influences from higher brain centres

Higher cortical influence

Pathology of the antero-medial parts of the frontal lobes gives rise to problems in micturition and defaecation, such as urgency, urge incontinence, loss of bladder sensation, and urinary retention. Other frontal lobe lesions produce social disinhibition and voiding at inappropriate times and places, although the voiding mechanism is normal.

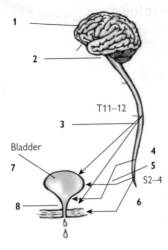

T11–12

Bladder

1. Frontal micturition area
2. Pontine micturition area
3. Thoracolumbar sympathetic chain
4. Onuf's nucleus
5. Parasympathetic nerves
6. Somatic pudendal nerve
7. Dettrusor muscle
8. External urethral sphincter

Fig. 7.1 Neural control of the bladder

Pathophysiology

Bladder and bowel disorders result from three levels of interruption (Table 7.1).
- Suprapontine.
- Suprasacral.
- Lower motor neuron.

Table 7.1 Pathophysiology of bladder and bowel disorders

Lesion	Functional change	Disease examples	Outcome
Suprapontine	Frontal lobe disconnection Periventricular demyelination Basal ganglia dysfunction Dilatation of lateral ventricle anterior horns	Brain injury Stroke MS Parkinson's disease	Hyper-reflexic bladder contractions Rarely, urinary retention
Suprasacral	Inhibition from medullary or spinal cord lesion Descending tracts lesions leads to incoordination of external sphincter and detrusor action	Spinal cord injury/ dysfunction, etc.	Hyper-reflexic bladder contractions producing urgency, frequency, urge incontinence Detrusor-sphincter dyssynergia
Lower motor neuron	S2/3/4 damage gives loss of bladder sensation Hypotonic bladder with relaxed external sphincter	Lumbar disc prolapse Trauma Intraspinal lesions	Urinary retention and leakage High residual volumes Stress incontinence

Bladder detrusor-sphincter dyssynergia

- This describes the failure of the sphincter to relax when the detrusor muscle contracts and is due to a spinal cord lesion causing incoordination governing external sphincter and detrusor muscle of the mechanism.
- It can give rise to raised intra-vesical pressure, upper tract dilatation, back pressure on kidneys, and renal damage.
- In addition, it can trigger distant problems in spinal cord injured patients with intact sensation with a consequent risk of hypertensive crises.
- Symptoms result in interrupted bursts of urinary flow between the detrusor forces expelling urine and the sphincter retaining urine.

Management of urinary problems

See Table 7.2 and Fig. 7.2.

Table 7.2 Management of urinary problems

Problem	Action	Reason
Impairment of renal function	Investigate (biochemical screen, ultrasound, IVU) and manage medical aspects	Need to preserve renal function for general health and life
Failure of bladder emptying	Assess post micturition volume by catheter drainage or ultrasound. >100mL significant	Residual urine stone formation, infection, renal dysfunction
	Involve continence nurse adviser—	
	Catheterization: intermittent	Intermittent catheterization carried out by individual or carer by clean rather than sterile technique using 8F or 10F catheter. At least twice daily. Best suited for people with functioning sphincters
	Catheterization: indwelling	Used when intermittent not possible. Size 14–16F silastic catheter. Suprapubic route is preferable in long term use because of better safety and urethral protection profiles.
	Treat any urinary infections	Protect renal function and general health
	Urinary retention (rare) due to poor detrusor contraction	Cholinergic, anti-cholinesterase or selective α-1 blocker medication
Detrusor hyper-reflexia	Cystometrogram	Assess intravesical pressure and detrusor hyper-reflexia
	Bladder training	Reduce intravesical pressure
	Anticholinergic medication	Reduce detrusor activity.
	Botulinum toxin	Intramuscular botulinum toxin has produced good results and lasts about 9 months. Injected via cystoscope.
	Catheter and condom drainage. Absorbent pads, napkins, etc	Protection against urinary leaking

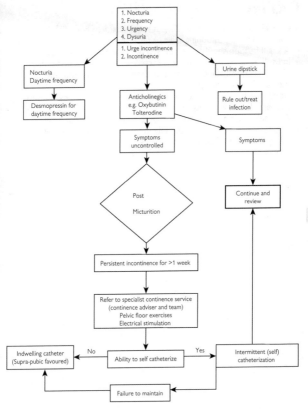

Fig. 7.2 Bladder management pathway

Catheters

- Intermittent catheters are safe, but require patient compliance and upper limb and positioning skills to perform.
- A small balloon should be employed to reduce nociceptive irritation. Indwelling catheters should be inserted under aseptic conditions.
- Complications include leakage, blockage, stone formation, infection, and the bladder constriction.
- Using larger catheters against leakage is erroneous, as they will simply increase detrusor irritability.
- Anticholinergic medication is useful to suppress detrusor activity.
- The suprapubic route is preferable in the long term due to better safety and urethral protection profiles.

Surgery

Please refer to a urology text for the indications and description of individual surgical procedures. Close working with a urology team is essential part of the rehabilitation team's work (📖 see Table 7.3).

Table 7.3 Surgical procedures

Procedure	Description
Sphincter ablation	Need decreased since use of botulinum toxin into detrusor muscle. Sphincterotomy rare now outside some spinal injuries units
Urinary diversions	Metrofanoff procedure—ileal conduit—allow good bladder control and change people's lives.
Other procedures	Clam cystoplasty Artificial urethral sphincters and sacral stimulators depend on an intact lower motor neuron—very effective, but require patient compliance 📖 see Fig. 7.3.

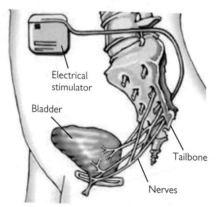

Electrical stimulator

Bladder

Tailbone

Nerves

Fig. 7.3 Anterior sacral stimulator (Bradley Scott)

Chapter 8

Sex and sexuality

General issues

Sex and sexuality are still among the most ignored and least discussed issues with people with disabilities. It is not actually known how many people report sexual dysfunction among the disabled population, but figures as high as 72% have been suggested. Professionals (even in rehabilitation settings) are often very embarrassed to talk about the subject and many still have an attitude that it is not a feature that is either worth mentioning or relevant to the lives of people with disabilities. There still persists today a feeling that disabled people should not have sexual feelings. The importance of sex and sexuality and discussing the emotional needs of disabled individuals and their families and carers are an essential part of discovering the whole person, whom one is trying to help.

Definitions

- Sexual function, taken outside the context of emotional needs, concentrates on physical function.
- Sexuality includes making relationships, the whole question of self-esteem, personal appearance and attraction to potential partners and is the very essence of the human spirit. It plays a full part in the lives of not only disabled people, but of the general population as well.

The desires and wishes for emotional and personal attachments among people with disabilities are no different from that of the rest of the population. They are often played down and it is known that people who have been disabled either from birth or from a very early age have decreased expectations. Their families also have decreased expectations and it is perhaps not surprising that many are scared or embarrassed to raise sex and sexuality as an issue. It is therefore important for the doctor or other members of the rehabilitation team to bring up the subject in an open and frank way, so that the whole subject can be discussed freely. There is often a huge relief of emotional frustration, once the individual can find an appropriate outlet for their feelings. Some psychosexual clinics have been established, but are still relatively uncommon. The teaching of sex and sexuality is now part of the curriculum for specialist trainees in Rehabilitation Medicine and concentrates on both the psychosocial aspects as well as the physical function. Techniques can be employed to assist function in the physical act and ensure satisfaction for the individual and for his or her partner, who may or may not be have a disability also. Some of these will be mentioned in the next section. Sexuality is more difficult to address and the whole idea of a man or woman with or without a physical disability discussing their sex life with a total stranger may fill many with dread. The experience, however, is often enlightening, but the individual should be given the opportunity to discuss this with whomsoever they like and it does not have to be a member of the rehabilitation team.

Common questions on functioning are:

- How might they be able to carry out intercourse while having a catheter in-situ?
- Will they have an episode of incontinence during intercourse, how will they physically get close enough to each other, and how might they relate a relationship to their friends and family?
- How will they deal with the prospect perhaps of pregnancy and parenthood?

Disabled people may well fail initially (just like most of the able-bodied population) but will need to persevere, to learn how to be intimate with their partners, without being overwhelmed by failing to match up to their own expectations.

Sexuality

While sex is the act of intimacy, sexuality is the persona of the individual, which attracts potential partners. As stated in 📖 General issues, p.120, disabled young people may be actively hindered in expressing their own sexual feelings and may not have had the freedom among their peers in the same way that able-bodied young people have. Very often, and particularly for young people, comfort with sexuality is as much a question of belonging to society as it an expression of what people want. Sexuality issues for people with acquired disabilities may also be different and a change in self-esteem is an important issue. Many men may be impotent and 80–90% of these are usually psychogenic. With time, relaxation, and confidence, impotence usually resolves, but there are always going to be a few who are going to need help to get over this problem. Again, as already discussed, sexual performance need not necessarily be considered as the only yardstick to measure satisfaction in personal relationships. The promotion of quality of life in an open and full relationship may be just as rewarding as the ability to carry out sexual intercourse.

Male sexual function

Impotence tends to be associated with lesions of the spinal cord or cauda equina. Involvement of the autonomic and sensory pathways may give rise to impaired erectile function in males, due to impaired vaso-congestion of the corpora cavernosa and spongiosa. The lower the level of the lesion, the more likely that impotence will be organic in nature. Those men with an intact sacral portion of the spinal cord are likely to achieve reflex erection, although this may be inadequate for intercourse. Overall, about half of spinal cord injured men have sufficient erection for intercourse. Sacral anterior stimulator implants can be used to achieve this.

Men with erectile dysfunction were historically managed by intra-cavernosal injections of papaverine, which could give rise to penile fibrosis, but the management of erectile dysfunction has now been superceded by drugs, such as sildenafil or tadalafil and second generation developments. Sildenafil, taken 1 hour or so before intercourse, is useful in allowing an appropriate development of an erection in response to a normal emotional stimulation. There is a dose-related response, but most people find that between 25mg and 100mg is sufficient with 50mg being the standard dose. It may give rise to coronary insufficiency and care should be taken in men as they get older. It is contra-indicated in established coronary artery disease. Alprostadil has been of interest in producing penile rigidity by local stimulation of the glans penis for men unable to take sildafenil. The drug is applied with an applicator and an erection may be expected within 15 minutes.

Ejaculatory function is affected more commonly than erectile function in spinal cord injured men. Only 5% of men with a complete upper motor neurone lesion and 18% with a complete lower motor neurone lesion report any persistence of the ability to achieve ejaculation. The treatment may consist of vibration applied to the penis with or without electrical stimulation, using a probe placed in the rectum. This can promote ejaculation by allowing the semen to be collected, but it has to be stated that these techniques are in the management of infertility in spinal cord injured patients rather than in the promotion of the sexual act. Electro-ejaculation is also possible in the clinic, but again this is for achievement of fertility. All vibration techniques are able to be used at home, but care is required in patients with an injury above the level of D6. Autonomic hyper-reflexia can occur with all its attendant problems. Management of urinary infections is obviously important as they will limit already impaired spermatogenesis. Similarly, older fashioned techniques, such as sphincterotomy, may result in retrograde ejaculation of semen and this procedure is finding less and less favour for many other reasons.

Female fertility

Many women with disabilities may have never received education on contraception or had much discussion on their own sexuality issues. While 75% of men report sexual dysfunction, it is less common in women at 56%. Many describe fatigue, diminished sensation, loss of libido, and orgasmic dysfunction. This is particularly evident in people with multiple sclerosis and traumatic brain injury. Hyposexuality is a common change after the latter, although disinhibition and hypersexuality have been reported following a frontal injury.

Pregnancy carries with it increased risks of, for instance, pressure sores and sepsis, particularly in the urinary tract. Antenatal care should be carried out in conjunction with a spinal injuries unit. Women with injuries at the D10 level or above are at risk of premature delivery and at D6 and above, of autonomic dysreflexia which is particularly evident as a warning of impending labour. Epidural anaesthesia should be considered as the method of choice for these particular women.

Chapter 9

Eating and swallowing disorders

Introduction

Swallowing disorders are common. Probably about half of people after a stroke have a swallowing disorder at some point during the recovery process and problems with swallowing are as common after traumatic brain injury, Parkinson's disease, and in the later stages of multiple sclerosis and motor neuron disease. A whole variety of other neurological problems such as myasthenia gravis and muscular dystrophies, as well as a range of local pathologies, such as mouth and laryngeal cancer, can also cause swallowing difficulties.

Swallowing is essential to maintain nutrition and to deal with saliva. About 1–1.5 litres of saliva are produced daily, which requires an awake adult to swallow about once per minute—around 1000 times per day plus the additional swallowing required during eating.

First it is important to recognize that a swallowing problem exists. Sometimes the problem is obvious and the person will volunteer a difficulty with chewing, swallowing, coughing, or spluttering during or soon after eating. However, occasionally the problem is less obvious, particularly in children or those with cognitive impairments. The clues in such individuals may be as follows:
- Recurrent chest infections.
- Weight loss.
- Malnutrition.
- Taking excessive time over food.
- Food residue in the mouth after eating.
- Excessive secretions.
- Wet or hoarse voice after food.
- Sensation of food sticking in the throat.
- Reflux or regurgitation of food or fluid.
- Difficulty breathing.
- Pain when swallowing.
- Laborious chewing.
- Increased throat clearing.
- Post-prandial wheezing.

Thus, there are many clues to eating and swallowing disorders for people who are not able to report difficulties themselves.

The recognition of such disorders is vital, as malnutrition and recurrent pneumonia commonly accompany recurrent swallowing problems. The advent of percutaneous endoscopic gastrostomy (PEG) feeding has now made the management of swallowing disorders much simpler once the diagnosis is made.

Assessment

The clinical assessment of dysphagia is a multidisciplinary process. There are now expert speech and language therapists who specialize in dysphagia management who will work in partnership with the dietician and physician—particularly a radiologist to undertake videofluoroscopic assessments and a surgeon to undertake insertion of PEG feeding tubes.

As in all branches of medicine it isimportant to first take a thorough clinical history. Not all problems with eating are associated with problems of swallowing. In some people difficulty with behaviour, mood, or cognition can all interfere with or prevent eating. People with a reduced level of alertness may have difficulty eating. After stroke, for example, severe problems of perception or dyspraxia can prevent the individual using plates and cutlery properly. They may not be able to see or recognize food or may be incapable of coordinating the necessary hand and mouth movements to eat and drink. There may be problems cutting up food or difficulty holding a cup because of severe tremor. Problems with receptive language can prevent someone from understanding instructions that 'dinner is ready'. An individual with severe depression may simply not wish to eat. Thus, a swallowing and nutritional assessment cannot be taken out of context from a general assessment of behaviour, mood, cognition, and intellect.

Nutritional assessment

Assessment should be made of the nutritional state. Body weight and height measurements can lead to a calculation of the surface area to weight ratio. Ideal ratios are known. Total body fat can be estimated by skin-fold measurements, such as the biceps, triceps, or iliac sites, and normal parameters are available. An accurate weight record is sometimes the only way to determine whether there is an ongoing nutritional or swallowing problem.

Examination of the oral cavity and tongue

The general condition of the mouth, teeth, and the fit of the dentures all need proper examination. There may be:
• Trauma, infection, or structural abnormality in the oral cavity.
• Impaired secretion of the salivary glands.
• Decayed or inadequate dentition or poorly fitting dentures.

All these features will obviously need different treatments in their own right.

Examination of swallowing

A limited amount of information can be obtained from observing a normal swallow. The individual should be alert and seated in an upright and symmetrical position. It is useful for the person to swallow water as well as food with a thick, smooth consistency, such as custard or yoghurt. The examiner should see if the larynx rises to indicate a swallow or if there are clinical signs of swallowing dysfunction such as coughing, spluttering, respiratory distress, or a wet, hoarse voice.

There is, however, only one proper way to assess swallowing and that is by use of a *videofluoroscopic swallowing examination*. This will allow assessment of swallowing function during all stages of the swallowing process. In most assessments a number of different food consistencies are given, such as barium liquid, barium mixed with yoghurt, and a barium cookie. The radiologist will screen the chewing and swallowing phases in order to make a diagnosis of the problem. Sometimes various manoeuvres can be tried out during the screening sessions that might improve the individual's swallowing function.

The commonest result of swallowing problems is misdirection of the food or fluids into the airway—known as *penetration*. The passage of food past the vocal cords into the trachea and beyond can cause varying degrees of respiratory discomfort or respiratory compromise. The extent to which inhaled food causes a problem will depend on the amount and frequency of the aspiration as well as the individual's own general condition. Some individuals seem to tolerate aspiration without problems but in most people aspiration is likely to lead to recurrent chest infections and pneumonia.

Finally it is important to note the presence of a *gag reflex* should *never* be taken as a sign of safe oral feeding.

Carer/feeder assessment

Sometimes an apparent eating or swallowing problem is not confirmed on examination and the difficulty is actually not a problem with the disabled person but with the carer or feeder. Time and care in food preparation is often required and considerable effort is sometimes needed in the feeding process. A child with cerebral palsy, for example, can take up to an hour to take an adequate meal. Rushed preparation and inappropriate attention to posture and to the likes and dislikes of the individual can all lead to problems.

Nerve supply

A number of cranial nerves are involved in the swallowing process
(see Table 9.1). Normal clinical examination of these cranial nerves is
an important part of the overall assessment of someone with swallowing
difficulties.

Table 9.1 Cranial nerves involved in the swallowing process

Cranial nerve	Function
V	Muscles of mastication and sensation to the anterior two-thirds of the tongue and buccal cavity
VII	Nerve to supply the orbicularis oris muscle required for lip closure and taste to the anterior two-thirds of the tongue
IX	Taste and sensation to the posterior third of the tongue and buccal cavity and sensation to the tonsils, laryngeal mucosa, and soft palate and involvement of the gag and cough reflexes
X	Similar to IX but also involved with phonation and vocal cord closure in the larynx and sensation and motility of the oesophagus
XII	Movement of the tongue

Normal swallowing mechanism

Swallowing is conveniently divided into four main stages:

- Stage 1—oral preparation. At this stage food is bitten, chewed, and masticated and compressed into a bolus. This phase will clearly rely on proper coordination of the lips, tongue, and jaw and will require an adequate quantity of saliva (Fig. 9.1a).
- Stage 2—oral phase. This stage involves the voluntary transfer of the bolus or fluid towards the pharynx. The tongue plays a major part in this process and will move the food bolus upwards and backwards to contact with the hard palate. When the bolus reaches the anterior faucial arch the reflex swallow is initiated (Fig. 9.1b, c).
- Stage 3—pharyngeal phase. This is a reflex stage and is no longer under voluntary control (Fig. 9.1d, e). This stage will involve a number of important muscular actions:
  - Closure of the velopharynx to prevent food and fluid refluxing into the nose.
  - Closure of the larynx to prevent material entering the larynx. This is achieved by laryngeal elevation and anterior movement which also has the effect of stretching and helping to open the cricopharyngeal muscle.
  - Peristalsis of the pharynx in order to help propel the bolus towards the oesophagus.
  - Opening of the cricopharyngeal muscle and passage of the bolus into the oesophagus.
- Stage 4—oesophageal phase. This is again an automatic stage involving passage of the bolus from the relaxed upper oesophageal sphincter at the level of the cricopharyngeal muscle down the oesophagus to enter the stomach through the relaxed gastro-oesophageal/cardiac sphincter (Fig. 9.1f).

It is important to emphasize that videofluoroscopy is the only way to obtain an accurate assessment of swallowing and a determination of the part of the swallowing process that is at fault.

Video recording is possible, which allows a more detailed analysis of the rapid automatic swallowing phases.

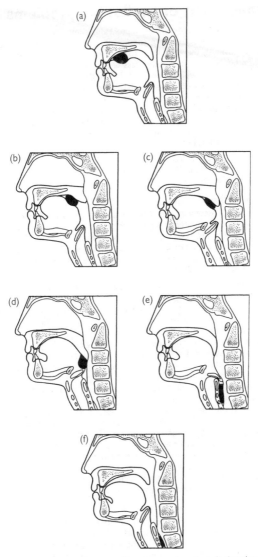

Fig. 9.1 The four stages of swallowing: (a) oral preparatory stage; (b, c) oral stage; (d, e) pharyngeal stage; (f) oesophageal stage

Management of swallowing problems

As with all parts of the rehabilitation process it is important that any treatment intervention is accurately monitored. Repeat videofluoroscopy may be used, but obviously there are limits to the number of times a videofluoroscopy can be repeated. Thus other less direct measures of monitoring are useful, such as regular monitoring of the weight. In particular calculation of the body mass index (BMI) is useful. This is calculated as the weight (in kg) divided by the height (in metres) squared. It is also useful to maintain an accurate diet history. This can include the details of the food and liquid intake as well as the consistency of the food, the number of times the individual coughs or splutters on food during a typical meal, and length of time taken to complete the meal, etc.

Next it is necessary to calculate energy and protein requirements so that the necessary dietary intake can be calculated. At this point involvement of a dietician becomes essential.

Modifying the oral diet

The videofluoroscopy may well have indicated the type of food consistency that is best tolerated. It is often the case that thin fluids, such as soup, or crumbling foods, such as biscuits, are best avoided. Usually smooth, semi-solids are best, which in turn requires thickened fluids or a pureed or soft diet. Once again advice from a dietician is necessary as such diets can be bland and disliked by the individual.

The videofluoroscopy may have indicated other possible compensatory strategies. Some general guidelines would include:

- Posture—variations to head and neck posture can sometimes alleviate a swallowing disorder and in any case, if at all possible, the head and neck should be upright and symmetrical.
- Learning to relax and not to talk during eating can be helpful.
- It is often useful to develop a feeding regimen that involves small amounts of food in the mouth with a quite clear deliberate chewing phase leading to a purposeful swallow.
- Generally several small meals a day are preferable to two or three big meals both from the point of view of the swallowing and to eliminate problems with fatigue—both in the disabled person and the carer.
- There is some evidence that exercises can improve oral motor control, strength, and range of movement and bolus control.
- There are some specific techniques for a delayed swallowing reflex. In such people the reflex is triggered too late to prevent some aspiration. In some cases stroking of the faucial arches with a cold laryngeal mirror prior to eating seems to trigger a reflex more effectively. Occasionally sucking on ice can have a similar effect.

Nutritional supplements

Nutritional supplements should be considered as soon as there is evidence that the dietary intake alone is insufficient. There is now a wide range of oral nutritional supplements and these are generally protein and energy dense and are also prescribable in a variety of flavours. There are also high-energy snacks, meals, and drinks that can supplement an inadequate diet.

Artificial nutritional support

When oral nutrition is contra-indicated because of the risk of aspiration or is inadequate to meet nutritional requirements then some form of non-oral feeding becomes necessary. There are basically two non-oral routes—nasogastric feeding and gastrostomy feeding.

Nasogastric feeding

Nasogastric feeding is quick to initiate and is often used in the early days after an acute event, such as a stroke or brain injury when the individual is unable to take any or little oral nutrition. There are now highly durable, fine-bore polyurethane tubes that are easy to insert and reasonably comfortable to have *in situ* for a few days. However, there are significant problems with nasogastric feeding. Many people find the tube uncomfortable. The tubes often need replacement and re-intubation can be upsetting as well as a potential cause of nasal trauma. Other disadvantages include blocking of the tube, displacement of the tube, and indeed the nasogastric tube itself might further impair a defective swallowing mechanism.

Percutaneous endoscopic gastrostomy

In recent years PEG feeding has gained wider acceptance as a quick and safe alternative to a surgical gastrostomy. There is no need for general anaesthesia and insertion of the tube is a simple procedure just requiring a local anaesthetic and sometimes a short-term intravenous sedative. There is a very low complication rate of <1%. Tubes can be placed under radiological direction or more commonly by assistance with an endoscope. The tubes are well tolerated and there is less risk of tubes becoming blocked or being dislodged.

Tube feeds can be administered either by bolus or by continuous pump. Sometimes overnight feeding via a pump is useful in supplementing an inadequate oral intake. However, for those who need most or all of their nutrition through the tube then bolus feeding is generally best as this has the advantage that the patient is free to be more mobile for large parts of the day. Usually boluses are administered at 4–6 hours or indeed at normal mealtimes. Usually people can tolerate 200–400ml of a feed at a time which will require just three to four feeds per day. Liquid medication can also be given down the tube.

Problems

Other than problems with the tube itself—such as blockage and dislodging—there are a number of common problems such as diarrhoea, abdominal pain, abdominal distension, gastric reflux, and vomiting. Sometimes it can be quite a long process to adjust the feeding regimen to reduce such symptoms to a minimum.

However, PEG feeding is usually easy and safe and is now widely practised for many people both in the short term following a recoverable condition, such as stroke or brain injury, or in the long term for those with permanent swallowing disorders, such as those with multiple sclerosis or motor neuron disease.

Further reading

1. Carrau RL and Murry T (1999). *Comprehensive management of swallowing disorders.* Plural Publishing, San Diego & Abingdon.
2. Jones B (2003). *Normal and abnormal swallowing: imaging in diagnosis and therapy,* 2nd edn. Springer-Verlag, New York.
3. 🖥 www.nlm.nih.gov/medlineplus/swallowingdisorders.html —a useful general guide to dysphagia and swallowing disorders produced by the National Institute for Neurological Disorders and Stroke, with references to other relevant web resources.

Chapter 10

Communication

Introduction and referral

Communication encompasses speech, non-verbal communication, special senses (the ability to hear and to see), and is reliant on normal cognitive function. Speech and language therapists have a major role to play in the assessment of communication and in the treatment of its disorders, but the whole rehabilitation team has to be skilled in recognizing and adopting the most effective and sensitive way to communicate with patients. People with communication disorders are frequently poorly appreciated and feel that it is the world at large that has the problem. Those with pure motor speech deficits however, usually understand that they have a problem and become immensely frustrated by it.

Assessment

Those whose communication interferes with their participation in society require an assessment from a speech and language therapist. Assessment may take quite a long time, even in skilled hands, and other professionals may not have the time or the expertise to make a thorough appreciation of the problems. Care should be given to ensuring that, at the time of referral, the patient can actually cope with and understand the assessment process. Speech and language therapists are concerned with all aspects of communication in terms of improving personal communication skills in general, including non-verbal communication, and can pass on that advice to the rest of the rehabilitation team. They can thus provide other team members and families with a consistent approach to patients to achieve an appropriate response or reply in order to reduce the frustration to a minimum.

Speech and language disorders

See Table 10.1 for descriptions of disorders.

Table 10.1 Speech and language disorders

Disorders	Descriptions
Disorders of speech	Speech or articulation depends on normal musculature. Loss of neuromuscular control of the structures involved in articulation results in slurring of speech, *dysarthric speech*.
	Tone and quality affected by damage to the tongue, the lips, the palate, the vocal cords, and lungs, e.g. in cleft palate's hypernasal sound.
	Damage to articulation can occur following resuscitation after a stroke or traumatic brain injury.
	Anarthria is used to describe complete loss of speech due to impairment of neuromuscular control.
Disorders of language	*Dysphasia* is characterized by four elements:
	Motor: *Sensory:* Expression Comprehension Writing Reading
	The cause of a motor loss is a lesion affecting the dominant hemisphere in the parietal and temporal areas. Reading and writing may also be affected, but receptive involvement suggests a more extensive lesion.
	Global dysphasia suggests impairment of all aspects of language and the patient may only be able to make unintelligible grunting sounds.
Disorders of fluency	*Stammering or stuttering* results from hesitations and blocking of speech and tends to be less common in adults. Chronic neurological disease (spinal cord injury and multiple sclerosis in particular) can produce intercostal and diaphragmatic muscle weakness, which reduces breath control and thus fluency.
Disorders of voice	*Dysphonia* may be organic or psychological. Polyps, nodules and oedema of the vocal cords cause abnormal stresses and tensions and are commonly found in singers.
	Although speech is usually intelligible, it is quite embarrassing for people, as it may affect the ability of people to regain work e.g. from local laryngeal damage in surgery.

Commonly associated diseases

Stroke (Table 10.2)

About 15% of stroke sufferers will have a significant dysphasia. Non-dominant parietal lobe lesions in stroke may give a transient dysarthria, which usually recovers well, but there may also be a loss of non-verbal communication.

Traumatic brain injury

Both dysphasia and dysarthria are seen, but often resolve quite quickly in contrast to stroke patients. The main communication difficulties lie in non-verbal communication and cognitive deficits and the speech and language therapist works with the rest of the rehabilitation team to find a consistent way to approach and communicate with the disabled individual.

Multiple sclerosis

Spastic and ataxic dysarthria may both occur with disease progression from difficulties around the tongue and mouth. As a result, feeding difficulties may occur.

Other chronic neurological diseases

Parkinson's disease, motor neuron disease, and myasthenia gravis all produce dysarthrias and dysphonias and patients with Parkinson's disease classically get quieter as the disease progresses. The on–off periods of disease control affects speech greatly and very often one can judge symptom control on speech alone.

Cerebral palsy

Communication is a major feature of assessment. Dysarthria and dysphonia are common, but language disorders are less common and are usually associated with learning disabilities. Signing systems such as hand signs, Makaton or Bliss signs can improve communication and the input of a speech and language therapist is very important here.

Table 10.2 Dysphasia

Dysphasia	Function	Site of lesion
Expression	Motor	Postero-superior temporal and frontal lobe lesions
Comprehension	Sensory	Postero-inferior temporal lobe lesions

Communication aids

Communication aids may be useful substitutes for verbal communication and may transform a person's life. They are indicated for severe dysarthria and expressive dysphasia, yet they may be quite simple. They tend to be less helpful where there is a receptive disorder. Users require considerable motivation, which rules out their use in some people with cognitive or learning difficulties 📖 see Table 10.3.

Table 10.3 Communication aids

Type of aid	Description
Direct select	Uses part of a body to indicate a symbol, e.g. Canon communication aid—a small hand held method of typing words for communication. The moderately intelligent person may prefer to use a word board, which points to the letters and some become very adept at writing out words.
Scanning	This method is chosen for people with very severe physical disabilities. A series of options comes up on a screen and the user can then point or signal the correct choice.
Encoding	Uses key symbol for the use of phrases, so pressing a certain symbol on the keyboard will produce a pre-set phrase and allow more fluent communication. May be used by cognitively intact people, who wish to use a relatively large vocabulary. Even though it may be limited shortly after the stroke, encoding methods are ambitious and can be combined with direct selection, scanning and environmental control equipment.

Patient follow-up

Follow up over many months and even years is essential, as recovery is slow. People may have to wait several years to see any significant improvements in expression after a stroke. Users of communication aids must be checked to make certain that they are using them correctly and that the aid is valuable to them in their everyday lives rather than just for therapy. Many find them vital for quality of life, but many also give them up because they can use non-verbal communication better to communicate with their friends and family. More extensive communication aids can be obtained from regional centres, such as Access to Communication Technology.

Chapter 11

Other physical problems

Introduction

This chapter will include some of the many physically disabling conditions, which do not conveniently fit into either diagnosis or impairment-based classifications, such as pressure sores, contractures, pain within the context of physical disability, and the chronic fatigue syndrome (ME, fibromyalgia, etc.)

Pressure sores

Definition

An area of erythema under the skin, which may progress to ulceration and subcutaneous tissue necrosis as a result of ischaemia due to unrelieved pressure. This is sometimes the result of shear forces on structures over bony points, which disrupts the circulation to deep tissues. This therefore causes an ischaemic injury, which results in tissue breakdown.

Features

- Pressure sores cause significant mortality and morbidity—95% of them are totally preventable and cause immense cost to health services. Even now, 3–11% of all patients admitted to hospital develop a pressure sore.
- Characterized initially by persistent skin erythema where pressure from friction forces injures blood vessels in the skin; this results in ischaemia, cell necrosis, and superficial ulceration.
- Deeper structures may be affected by shear forces occurring in the neighbourhood of bony prominences, which give rise to more extensive subcutaneous destruction through damage to subcutaneous blood vessels.
- The necrotic tissue invariably becomes infected, causing inflammation of surrounding tissues and systemic toxicity.
- Maceration of the skin by sweat and urine reduces its tensile strength and the elderly are at special risk because of a decrease in the skin's tolerance to stress, which increases the likelihood of breakdown.

See Table 11.1 for clinical features and stages.

Table 11.1 Clinical features and staging

Stage	Feature
1. Discoloration of intact skin including non-blanchable erythema or loss of epidermis.	Starts at surface and progresses inwards.
2. Partial skin loss involving epidermis and dermis.	Heals within weeks
3. Full thickness skin loss extending to subcutaneous tissues	Starts deep and causes skin necrosis from below. Takes months to heal.
4. Full thickness skin loss with extensive destruction involving muscle and bone and other deep structures with tissue necrosis.	

Who is at risk?

Patients experiencing:

- Immobility through neurological disease, especially:
  - Tetra/paraplegia.
  - Obesity.
  - Coma/confusion.

- Sensory loss due to:
  - Severe physical disease.
  - Weight loss.
  - Low albumin.
  - Low vitamin C.
- Deformity:
  - Producing abnormal loads.
  - From fractures.
  - From spasticity due to faecal and urinary incontinence.

Prevention

- Use of Norton or Waterlow Scale[1,2].
- Identification and education of 'at risk' patients.
- Management of deformities and 2–3 hourly turning in chair and bed.
- Seating, cushions, and mattresses.

Management (Table 11.2)

Table 11.2 Management of pressure sores

Physical measures	Relief of pressure is the most important factor
	Debridement of necrotic tissue—can be done on ward in insensate patients, speeds up healing process
General health	Good diet containing protein and vitamin C is essential
	Adequate fluid intake
	Haematinics to treat anaemia
	Ensure patient can maintain Hb of >10g/dL
	Treatment of constipation/faecal loading
	Prevention of urinary/faecal incontinence
Topical treatments	Semi-permeable films to cover ulcers and soothe the skin
	Antiseptic agents to reduce infection
	Alginate dressings/hydrocolloid/hydrogel systems to absorb exudate
	Enzymes, hydrocolloid and hydrogel systems to remove slough
	Agents to promote granulation tissue
Infection	Antibiotics necessary for deep sores and for underlying bone infection
Surgery (adjunct to conservative therapy only)	Primary repair
	Formal plastic and reconstructive surgery—to provide skin and muscle flaps for weight-bearing areas (buttock, sacrum, trochanter), as a graft will often not survive the stresses and strains

References

1. Norton D (1961). Preventing pressure sores of heels. *Nursing Times*, **57**, 695–6.
2. Waterlow J (1985). Pressure sores: a risk assessment card. *Nursing Times*, **81**, 49–55.

Contractures

Definition

Restriction of limb movement leading to loss of function (dexterity, mobility etc.).

Features

Tendon and joint contracture occurs in prolonged immobility, due to either neurological or musculo-skeletal pathology. Muscle and tendon shortening or joint capsule restriction occurs leading to fibrosis and loss of range of movement across articulations and limbs. The process may start as a result of pain in a limb, joint disease, spasticity, or simple poor positioning. As a result, considerable time and effort must be spent in stretching the limbs in order to reverse the process and contractures lead to severe problems, such as pain, perineal hygiene, inability to place the foot flat on the ground, loss of dexterity and notably, poor self-esteem, and mood changes.

Treatment

Unchanged over years. Difficult and often painful, but where contractures are established, serial splinting and/or surgery should be considered.
- *Serial splinting*—the limb is stretched and a resin cast is applied, which is left for 7–10 days and then removed. The limb is then stretched further and a new cast is applied. Very often, back slabs or univalved cylinders are used to facilitate inspection of the limb and allow physiotherapy.
- *Surgery*—where return of limb function is not possible, as in patients with severe hemiplegia or paraplegia, tenotomy or arthrotomy operations may be needed to allow tissue release and further stretching is applied.

Chronic pain

This describes a condition, where the emotional elements account for a significant part of the syndrome and have to be addressed if the pain is to be managed satisfactorily.

Common associated conditions
- Chronic musculoskeletal pain, e.g. neck and back pain.
- Central pain syndromes.
- Occupational upper limb disorders.
- Degenerative joint disease.
- Chronic regional pain syndrome (types 1 and 2).

Central pain syndromes

Thalamic pain following stroke or traumatic brain injury is disabling and can lead to dysaesthesia or an awareness of abnormal sensation in the affected area of the body, very often down one side. Disordered function of the spino-thalamo-cortical pathway, which is responsible for pain and temperature is thought to be the cause. Patients can often experience more than one type of pain. Movement, touch, cold, especially a cold breeze, can often bring on the pain.

Management

Start with anti-convulsants (in particular pregabalin, gabapentin, carbamazepine,). If no help, try tricyclic anti-depressant medication, muscle relaxants or even chlorpromazine. None has been validated for this and none are routinely successful.

Chronic regional pain syndromes (CRPS)

This is a group of disorders in which an injury or insult proximally can lead to pain distally in the limb. There are two types:
- Type 1—associated.
- Type 2—referred pain similar to type 1, but follows the course of a peripheral nerve.

Type 1
- This pain is continuous in nature and is accompanied by hyperalgesia and allodynia.
- Local abnormal sympathetic activity is observed, with changes in temperature and colour of the limb and abnormal sweating. The affected part becomes cold, pale and muscles become wasted.
- Contractures and osteopenia appear, giving the original name of Sudek's atrophy.
- Sympathetic blockade is the treatment of choice, which should be combined with active exercise and physiotherapy.
- Other measures for chronic pain relief, such as anti-depressant medication may be required.

Type 2
- The pain is also continuous in character, but is often described as burning in quality.
- It is confined to a nerve's distribution and may be associated with a peripheral neuropathy.

Management of pain

A thorough assessment of the patient and carer is required. Where patients have been complaining of pain for years from degenerative disease, further medical intervention may be inappropriate and this should be clearly communicated. However, painful exacerbations need to be treated with effective medication and mild, but active, exercise.

Patients should be responsible for their own management and should seek medical assistance only when initial measures have failed. Successful management is critically dependent on finding a regimen of treatment which will help the patient. A combined approach of physical exercise, medication, and other therapies is required for most patients. Cognitive behavioural therapy is effective at dealing with the overall issues surrounding the pain and the evidence points to its early use (📖 see Cognitive behavioural therapy, p.163).

Physical treatments and exercise

Prolonged physiotherapy for people with chronic pain increases dependence on health professionals and does not give better outcomes. Patients should be taught an exercise programme that encompasses general exercise to improve fitness, specific exercises to protect the affected part of the body, and information on how to deal with painful exacerbations. Manipulation and mobilization may be useful for this and for reducing muscle spasm and pain in acute situations, but there is no evidence that they or other treatments alter the natural history of chronic pain.

Transcutaneous nerve stimulation (TENS) or acupuncture are effective in reducing pain and can be used in combination with other treatments. They require suitable education to ensure their efficacy. Splints, corsets, and braces can be helpful for acute exacerbations, but long-term use leads to disuse muscle atrophy and should be avoided.

Medication (Table 11.3)

Table 11.3 Medications for chronic pain

Centrally-acting analgesics	Start with simple medication and increase the dose and the potency of opioid analgesics. Narcotic analgesics suppress natural endorphine production and can cause dependence, which is difficult to deal with. They thus have no real place in the management of chronic pain
Anti-depressants	Tricyclics are useful in treating anxiety and depression in chronic pain and probably have a synergistic action with analgesics. They should be used for periods of 3–6 months, as shorter periods of time are often ineffective
	Both tricyclic anti-depressants and selective serotonin re-uptake inhibitors (SSRIs) have an equal impact on pain relief, although some examples in these groups have a better action than others. Paroxetine tends to be more helpful in this situation than other SSRIs for its greater anxiolytic action. Taking amitriptyline and dosulepin at night helps to induce sleep, allowing a reasonable period of rest for the patient to be more resilient to cope with the following day
Muscle relaxants	Little role in the treatment of chronic pain. Short courses of diazepam are attempted for up to 10 days to deal with marked anxiety and muscle spasm
	Baclofen and dantrolene sodium are also sometimes used for their antispasm qualities in similar way, but caution should be applied to benzodiazepines, as they are associated with considerable side effects and dependence and their long-term use is not recommended

Specific injections (Table 11.3)

Table 11.3 Injections for chronic pain

Local injections	Corticosteroids into joints can be helpful in reducing active synovitis, even in the absence of overt inflammation
Local nerve blocks	Relieve pain in a multitude of conditions ranging from soft tissue problems to intractable pain from osteoarthritis, e.g. suprascapular nerve blocks for intractable shoulder pain
	Regional sympathetic blockade is used for many conditions, ranging from inflammatory joint disease and osteoarthritis to CRPS type 1. Although the effects are sometimes short-lived, the procedure is relatively straightforward. Even more simple is guanethidine blockade of distal limbs, using 20mg of guanethidine intravenously in a cuffed limb
Epidural injections	Useful for acute and acute intermittent relief of limb pain
	Long-term relief not demonstrated in chronic situations
Facet joint injection	Used in the facet joint syndrome and in lumbar spondylosis, although the evidence does not tend to support this in patient populations. It is probably of value in very specific patients, in whom there is referred pain and localized tenderness over one specific joint. Can allow relief of pain for several weeks, if not months.

Cognitive behavioural therapy

This involves developing certain behavioural characteristics to try to normalize activities in chronic pain. The patient is encouraged to attempt certain key tasks every day and follows this up with rest and evaluation of the pain level. It has had an effect in many patients and the aim is to develop a coping strategy to participation in day-to-day activities. Time is of the essence here and consistency of approach results in a better response. Evidence of its effectiveness has now been shown.[1,2]

Chronic fatigue syndrome (CFS)/fibromyalgia

📖 This subject will be addressed in Chapter 23.

References

1. Scheeres K, Wensing M, Knoop H, et al. (2008). Implementing cognitive behavioral therapy for chronic fatigue syndrome in a mental health center: a benchmarking evaluation. *Journal of Consulting & Clinical Psychology*, 76, 163–71.
2. Carville SF, Arendt-Nielsen S, Bliddal H, et al. and EULAR (2008). EULAR evidence-based recommendations for the management of fibromyalgia syndrome. *Annals of the Rheumatic Diseases*, 67, 536–41.

Chapter 12

Technical aids and assistive technology

Introduction

Technical aids cover all equipment for disabled people, whether for use in the home, at work or in the community at large. They range from simple devices in the kitchen or bathroom, to hoists, stair-lifts, and any item which may improve the standard of living for a disabled person. They are designed for use by either the subject themselves or to be operated by carers in their caring role. Occupational therapists have particular skills in this field and equipment can be viewed and inspected in disabled living centres (contact information through the Disabled Living Foundation[1]). Care equipment helps disabled people, but is also designed to protect their carers from injury, e.g. hoists protect carers from back pain. 📖 See Table 12.1.

Assistive technology encompasses any technical equipment to improve participation and independence among disabled people. It covers simple technical aids and any device—electronic or other—which the disabled person may operate within their homes or outdoors. See Table 12.1; 📖 also see Communication aids, p.150.

Table 12.1 Common technical aids

Location	Self use	Carer use
In bed	Electric bed adjustment	Draw sheets for turning
Transfers	Grab rails	Electric hoists
	Sliding boards	Standing hoists and frames
Bathroom	Shower equipment	Glideabout chairs
	Shower seat	Bath hoists
	Bath aids	
Independence at home	Environmental controls—📖 see Environmental control systems, p.180	Switches, etc.
	Remote controls for TV, radio, etc.	
Mobility	Wheelchairs and mobility aids	Assistant controlled wheelchairs
	Buggies, etc.	
Communication	Letter/word boards	Assist with aids—📖 see Communication aids, p.150
	Communication aids	

References
1. Disabled Living Foundation ⁂ www.dlf.org.uk/

Wheelchairs

Wheelchairs can be obtained either through the National Health Service (NHS) for people with long-term needs, or can be bought privately. Disabled people have identified specific needs and may require more than one wheelchair—for work, at college, and at home and services therefore have to be flexible and sensitive to these needs.

Considerations in wheelchair prescription

- Diagnosis—affects usage of the chair, the need for review and on the speed of delivery, e.g. in MND. Presence of complicating factors, e.g. spasticity.
- Frequency and intensity of chair usage during the day.
- Where will the chair be used? Local environmental factors:
  - Community—?outdoors.
  - Within the home only?
  - Both?
- Transfers in and out of the chair—unaided, standing, sideways, assisted by carer, transfer boards etc. Should arm rests be removable to allow sideways transfer?
- Transportation of chair.
- Needs of carer.
- Seating—need for cushion, special seating, or complex seating system, activities in the chair, other factors e.g. incontinence.

Types of wheelchair

- Push-chair/buggy:
  - Disabled children—similar features to those found for young able-bodied children.
  - Need to be supportive but easy to use, and should be able to fold away.
- Manual self-propelled—9 series wheelchairs; same sizes as 8 series, but have four small wheels.
- Attendant-propelled—8L standard 16" (~40cm) seat (seat widths up to 20" (~51cm)); 8BL has a 15" × 16" (~38 × 40cm) seat.
- Powered—indoor and indoor/outdoor use.

Many models and variations are now available. Attachments include trunk supports, altered armrests, tilting backrests, head supports, and adjustable footrests. More sporty wheelchairs are also now available through NHS provision, which have a greater 'street credibility' amongst the young. Lightweight wheelchairs sacrifice stability for weight. They thus have to have a rigid frame, which prevents them folding. Powered chairs also do not usually fold. Tetraplegics above the level of C5 may require an electric wheelchair. They are controlled by a joystick on a control box, but some patients may need a chin control, a blow and suck control, a head control, or even a photo-electric cell.

Getting a wheelchair is usually through a loan system, but some patients may use a voucher scheme, which covers their equipment up to a certain financial allowance. They can add to this through their own means.

Special seating

Definition (Table 12.2)

Special seating is that component of a seating system in either a static chair or a wheelchair, which is specifically prescribed for disabled people to accommodate or to control any postural difficulties or to manage problems that may arise from abnormal pressures due to deformity.

Table 12.2 Definitions for special seating criteria

Moderate disability	Good head control
	Good to fair trunk control
	May be unstable when sitting unsupported
	Good functional ability with minimal support on a stable base.
Mild disability	Good head control but poor trunk control
	Unable to sit in a stable position without support
	Limited hand control when sitting in a stable position
Severe disability	Poor head and trunk control
	Unable to sit without support
	Limited upper limb function
	Spinal curvature and joint contractures
Static support	Fixed skeletal deformity and pressure problems
	Maintains function and prevents deformities from worsening }a hybrid of } the two
Dynamic support	Enhances function } roles
	For weakness and motor impairment

Aims of special seating systems

- Achieves stability and balance.
- Reduces the effort to maintain posture.
- Prevents or delays the onset or worsening of deformities.
- Optimizes function.
- Provide comfort.
- Allows distribution of load to provide maximal pressure relief.
- Decreases cardiorespiratory burden through functional support.

The seating system depends on the severity of the disability, the abilities and requirements of the disabled person, and the ability and needs of carers and other environmental factors. Many systems are designed for children with multiple disabilities, including learning difficulties, who may have fixed deformities as a result of poor positioning in early life. An appropriate seating system can improve people's lifestyle and self-esteem.

A good seating system therefore should aim to:
- Enable good positioning for comfortable sitting, feeding, swallowing and communication.
- Encourage bladder and bowel drainage and function.
- Provide good eye contact.
- Support the trunk to decrease the effort of breathing.
- Provide comfort
- Be practical for carer function

Organization of services

Special seating systems are expensive and, in the context of health care constraints, cannot be freely available, unless there is a clinical need. Simpler seating systems are prescribed by local wheelchair services, but more complex equipment is provided by regional centres. The expertise there, from rehabilitation engineers, rehabilitation physicians, and specialized therapists, ensures a more cost-effective service provision. It is not within the remit of this book to go into the various models in any depth.

Footwear and orthoses

Orthoses are devices worn outside the body, which support and aid the function of that part (Box 12.1). All doctors and therapists acquire a basic training in orthotics at both undergraduate and postgraduate level in order to realise their potential value. As with other technical assistance, the decision to use an orthosis should be made after team discussion. The team should include a doctor, a therapist, nursing staff, and orthotists and each orthosis should be prescribed with a specific aim. Both the orthotist and patient should have a thorough knowledge of what the orthosis is attempting to do. If a device is not worn, then the whole process fails and the technical merits of the appliance serve no useful purpose. The team should thus estimate the patient's compliance and education is an important feature.

> **Box 12.1 Types of orthoses**
>
> - *Footwear*—insoles, shoe modifications, bespoke shoes.
> - *Supports*—collars, lumbar supports/belts, epicondylitis clasps.
> - *Splints*—static/resting (prevents movement and supports joints) or working/lively (helps to increase limb function).

Footwear

Foot pain is common and may be due to joint disease or to nerve injury from unsupported weight-bearing structures. Prevention of subtalar subluxation is important in established inflammatory joint disease in order to prevent pain distally and the wearing of good footwear is a cheap and effective way to help this. Many doctors do not realise how prescribing comfortable shoes can transform the lives of people with painful feet. The development of depth shoes has increased the range available and there is now less need for individually made (bespoke) surgical shoes.

Insoles

- *Medial longitudinal*—used for simple flat feet and for lateral plantar nerve compression.
- *Arch supports*—prevention of subtalar valgus subluxation, as found in rheumatoid and osteoarthritis.
- *Metatarsal domes*—transfer weight away from the metatarsal heads to the metatarsal shafts to relieve the pain from metatarso-phalangeal joint disease and subluxation. A larger size of shoe may be needed to prevent callosities on the dorsum of the toes and plastazote temporary domes should first be fitted to test their efficacy.
- *Heel insoles*—for traumatic heel and leg pain and plantar fasciitis. New materials using shock-absorbing pads are useful in preventing heel pain, e.g. Sorbothane® and Viscolast®.

Modified shoes

- *Shoe raises*—these are used to correct unequal leg lengths. The same leg length is not required to achieve a normal swing phase in walking and raising the sole by half the leg length difference works. Differences of <1cm are probably not worth correcting in this way.

- *Depth shoes*—these are enhanced footwear for people with deformed feet. They are lightweight with a non-slip sole and have a wide opening to allow easy fitting. They are fairly cheap to produce and cater for most deformities, and sufficient space is available to fit an insole. However, this should be checked first.
- *Bespoke shoes*—individually designed to fit people with difficult feet, and can fulfil a variety of functions from tough working shoes to comfortable lightweight items. They are expensive to make and casts of the foot are made before the final shoe is manufactured. The lengthy time taken in fitting contributes to their high cost.

Supports
- *Collars*—they support the neck and reduce pain, but do not truly prevent movement. For really effective immobilization of the head, skull, or halo, traction should be used. They reduce muscle spasm in the first few days following neck injury and patients with rheumatoid disease should be fitted with one prior to anaesthetic intubation to highlight caution during cervical spine extension manoeuvres.
- *Corsets*—the commonest indication is an acute lumbar disc protrusion with muscle spasm and support the anterior abdominal wall. Polythene jackets are used with variable success for the pain of osteoporotic vertebral collapse and to prevent the effects on respiration of increasing truncal weakness as seen in muscular dystrophies etc.
- *Epicondylitis clasps*—worn on the proximal forearm to decrease the load on the extensor and flexor muscle origins and tennis and golfer's elbow respectively; they transfer the effective origin point of the muscle to a point under the clasp through a tight grip over the muscle's belly and allow work or playing games.

Splints
- Functions:
  - Stabilize joints.
  - Reduce pain and inflammation through immobilization.
  - Place limb in the best functional position.
  - Protect joints leading to confident usage.
  - Prevent or reduce further deformity.
- Resting splints:
  - Immobilize the affected part of the limb.
  - Often used at night to rest joints.
  - Help may be required to apply and remove them, particularly if bilateral.
  - Example: a paddle splint for the wrist and hand for patients with rheumatoid arthritis.
- Working or lively splints:
  - Allow a limb to work in some functional way and may incorporate a moving part.
  - Either free-moving or against resistance.
  - Stabilizing one joint may result in better functional use of the whole limb.
  - Example: hand splint in radial nerve injury.

- Serial splinting:
  - Used to increase the range of joint movement to reduce joint or tendon limb contracture.
  - Will reduce even very large contractures, when accompanied by active physical treatment.
  - The limb is straightened to a comfortable maximum and the splint is applied.
  - The splint is then changed every 7–10 days to allow a straighter cast to be applied until the objective is achieved.

Types of splints

- *Resting splints*—made of orthoplast and used to relieve acutely inflamed joints. Useful as night resting splints and the wrist should be held in 10° of extension when they are applied.
- *Working wrist splints*—the Futuro® wrist splint is probably the best known in the UK. There is a metal bar on the volar surface, resting the wrist, but full use of the hand is allowed. The splint is used in carpal tunnel syndrome and in inflammatory arthritis. It is also prescribed in people with repetitive strain disorder, but its use here is probably unwise. An individually made orthoplast or polythene splint may be necessary if the wrist is deformed.
- *Working hand splints*:
  - E.g. indicated for extensor tendon rupture to preserve function function.
  - An opponens splint is used for painful first carpo-metacarpal joint in osteoarthritis.
- *Knee splints*—stabilize knees with collateral ligament or cruciate ligament dysfunction.

Ankle/foot orthoses

- Indicated for foot drop following lateral popliteal nerve palsy, L5 nerve root compression and stroke.
- Supports ankle and subtalar joint instability and may incorporate insole corrections.
- Made of lightweight ortholon, which is not particularly strong and cracks.
- A leg iron caliper, fixed to the heel of the shoe from a strap at the upper calf, may then be required.

How to get an orthosis

Footwear and orthoses can be obtained through the Orthotics Department in most hospitals and qualified orthotists are found there. Clear benefits to patients will occur if clinicians and orthotists together plan the indications and applications of orthoses for disabled people.

Table 12.3 Orthoses for knee conditions

Mild collateral ligament injuries	A simple knee corset (e.g. neoprene) allows the patient to exercise quadriceps and hamstring muscles.
More severe collateral ligament injuries	Full knee hinged corset for deformities of <20°
	Little is of help for deformities of >20°
Cruciate ligament injuries	More complex stabilization from brace to prevent antero-posterior movement.
Disrupted knees	Straight leg polythene jackets

Prostheses

Definition

Prostheses are devices which are often implanted and which aim to substitute the control of bodily functions, which have been impaired by disease, damage, or loss. The major prostheses encountered in rehabilitation refer to artificial limbs, joint replacement, and true implanted neurological prostheses.

Joint prostheses

Joint arthroplasty has revolutionized the management of chronic joint disease. Patients can now live their lives without pain and can virtually forget the severe disability, to which they were formerly subjected by their arthritis. It is useful in both degenerative (osteoarthritis) and inflammatory joint disease and most experience has been gained from hip replacement. The use of superior techniques and materials has allowed greater survival of the prosthesis and one can now expect a hip arthroplasty to last for 10–15 years. Results tend to be better in osteoarthritis than in rheumatoid arthritis as bone quality and the integrity of surrounding structures are more likely to be reserved. Reference to an orthopaedic or rheumatology textbook is recommended for further reading, but indications for surgery include nocturnal pain, loss of range of joint movement—such that function is impaired—progression of the underlying disease, and failure to respond adequately to medication and to physical treatment. Joint instability is not a contra-indication, but is likely to lead to a less favourable outcome if there is a significant deformity.

Various designs of the prosthesis are now available and surgery can replace either the whole joint or part of it. Many arthroplasty prostheses are now made of a mixture of metal and plastic to reduce load and give longer life. Revision is possible if and when the prosthesis loosens, but requires great care in order to give the new artificial joint as much chance as possible of being as successful as the first.

The major concern to arthroplasty operations is infection and pain in a replaced joint should alert the physician to the presence of either infection or loosening of the prosthesis. Radiographs tend not to be of much help, but occasionally sclerosis around the root of the prosthesis can indicate loosening. The investigation of choice is an isotope bone scan using technetium-99, which shows the characteristic features of loosening. If infection is suspected, gamma scanning with gallium or indium-labelled white cells can differentiate between acute and chronic inflammation. Gallium highlights lymphocytes, whereas indium targets polymorphonuclear white cells and both are thus of great help. Infection requires prolonged antibiotic therapy for at least 6–12 weeks and may necessitate the removal of the prosthesis. The surgeon will have to be confident that infection has been eradicated before considering a new prosthesis.

Neuroprostheses

These deal with implantable devices which aim to improve functional independence and quality of life in people impaired by neurological disease, damage, or loss. They are not commonly used and therefore patients' relatives, carers, and rehabilitation professionals need to know what such devices can and cannot do. In addition, the latter need to have an understanding of the range of patients who may potentially benefit from their use. Neuroprostheses can be divided into three broad groups which:

- Substitute for lost sensory functions (sensory prostheses).
- Substitute for lost motor functions (motor prostheses).
- Regulate deranged sensory or motor functions (neuromodulators).

Prostheses can result in either functional neurostimulation or functional substitution. The former differs in the time domain from all other forms of medical or surgical treatment and its impact on sensory or motor function can be controlled according to the functional requirements of the moment. At present, neurostimulation is fairly crude compared to that generated by the nervous system, but is improving all the time. A report on neuroprostheses and rehabilitation has been published by the British Society of Rehabilitation Medicine.[1] Neuroprostheses may for instance be able to help people considerably but does not alter the underlying impairment. It reduces disability but is not a substitute for active rehabilitation. Rehabilitation is also about education and the application of neuroprostheses must be accompanied by an educational process in their use and function. These devices are uncommon and therefore their prescription and fitting are limited to specialized centres. However, doctors referring into these centres should be certain that the present disabilities are unsatisfactorily managed and that the doctor, the patient, and the family agree that there is potential for further improvement with the use of an implant. Considerable motivation is required by some patients to gain anticipated benefits. Table 12.4 is a list of some of the devices available (after Rushton[1])

Table 12.4 Implanted neuroprostheses

106–106	In use in most countries, many centres:
	Cardiac pacemakers—for cardiac arrhythmias
	CSF shunts—for hydrocephalus
103–104	In use in several countries, specialized centres:
	Spinal dorsal column stimulator—usually for pain
	Phrenic stimulators—for ventilation
	Cochlear stimulators—for profound deafness
	Baclofen pumps—for spasticity
	Bladder controllers—for continence and voiding
102–103	Establishing a clinical role, more than one centre:
	Cerebellar stimulators—for spasticity, usually cerebral palsy
	Peroneal braces—for central foot-drop
	Activated gracilis slings—for ano-rectal incontinence
	Upper limb stimulators—for grasps in C5/6 quadriplegia
102–103	Investigational devices:
	Lower limb stimulators—for paraplegic standing or walking
	Cerebellar stimulators—for epilepsy
	Visual cortex stimulators—for blindness
	Deep brain stimulators—for pain, tremor or movement disorders
	Cavernosal drug pumps—for impotence

References

1. Rushton DN (ed.) (1997). British Society for Rehabilitation Medicine. *Neuroprostheses, neuro-modulators, and rehabilitation medicine*. British Society for Rehabilitation Medicine, London.

Environmental control systems

One of the greatest benefits that modern technology has brought to the lives of disabled people is the ability to control their own lives at home. Opening the door to a caller, closing curtains, switching channels on TV or radio seem such commonplace activities for able-bodied people, but an inability to do this can be very frustrating for disabled people. Furthermore, their carers are tied to the house and safety worries exist. Environmental control systems (ECSs) can change all this by providing a means for a person with a severe physical disability to control the access to their her home, to summon emergency help, to operate everyday appliances such as the telephone, television etc., and to switch on and off electrical power for lighting and for other pieces of equipment. Increasing independence at home means that a disabled person can do much more of what they wish in safety, thereby leaving carers free to leave the house to gain much needed respite, as well as to do the shopping, etc.

Environmental control equipment has itself considerably advanced technologically and visual display units are now commonplace. The use of radiowaves and infra-red has meant that direct electrical wiring linkages between the control box and the target appliances have now disappeared, making the home much safer for the disabled individual and for carers. No longer do people have to worry about tripping over wires etc. In addition, whereas separate switches were required for able-bodied members of the household, this is no longer the case and they can now operate the same appliances as the disabled person, which allows better integration for all concerned.

Organizational arrangements

ECSs are provided through regional centres in most parts of the country. A regional ECS coordinator is appointed to link in and liaise with local coordinators in each health district (usually occupational therapists working within a rehabilitation centre). The regional coordinator is also responsible for training, budget management, contract negotiation, supply and maintenance of equipment, and maintenance of the contract database. The local coordinator, on the other hand, is tasked with patient follow-up, maintaining contract standards and local databases and local liaison between users and professionals.

So how do disabled people get ECSs? Firstly, their attending professionals must have the training to have them in mind and know how they may be useful for a particular disabled individual. After the completed referral form is sent to the regional coordinator, a medical assessment is undertaken by a trained assessor, usually a consultant in Rehabilitation Medicine. The assessment includes the individual's other needs, as well as that of the environmental control system. The assessor reports back to the regional coordinator with detailed recommendations of the needs of the disabled individual and of potential solutions in the form of environmental control equipment. The client is then seen by the local coordinator, who is thereafter responsible for provision of equipment and coordination of delivery. Rehabilitation engineers assess the interface between the patient and the equipment within the home and the local coordinator will follow the individual up. Although ECSs are provided through the health budget, the wiring and any adaptations to the house require Social Services approval and funding and thus their community occupational therapists also play an important role.

The equipment

ECSs usually comprise three different components:

- The selection unit, which acts as a nerve centre for the system.
- The input from the user to control the selection or new settings for various appliances.
- Commands to the controlled appliances.

Typical control appliances would be a door entry phone with an alarm or intercom system, light switches, telephone dialling systems, radio/TV/home entertainment control switches and on and off facility. Curtains and doors can also be opened and closed, but are usually extra items. The switches to control systems may be operated from a wheelchair or from a static surface and various types are available. These include a hand-operated lever or joystick, a chin or headrest switch, suck and puff and pressure pad switches, as well as specialized inputs for picking up eye movements. The Fox environmental control (RSL Steeper Ltd.) and Companion environmental control (Possum Controls Ltd.) are some of the latest available models, but there are many older ones still in service, which their users find more than satisfactory.

The assessment process

What should the assessment include? The medical history and its relevance to the assessment and the cause and progress of the disabling condition are, of course, important. The 24-hour care profile and the hours in which a disabled person is to be left unattended must be documented. Many severely disabled people are not in fact left very much by their carers and this may be for two reasons. The first is that they do not actually wish to be left unattended and the second is that the carers are fearful of going out. Obviously, these aspects need to be tackled sensitively, but, in these circumstances an environmental control may not be very useful and may end up as yet another piece of unused equipment in the house. In addition, opportunities for socializing are important and may require inclusion in the assessment.

The health and needs of the carers require documentation, along with their burden of care and any physical or lifestyle restrictions they may have. The examination should not only include the individual's motor function, but their mental state, cognitive abilities and their special senses (vision and hearing). It is obviously important that they can see the screen or listen to the bleep sounds. Surveying the environment will inform the assessor of other pieces of equipment currently in use. Unmet needs, both social and practical, also require documentation. Armed with this information, the assessment can then recommend a particular system and a trial may be necessary in order to identify whether or not the equipment is actually appropriate and of value.

Driving

Independent mobility has transformed the lives of some disabled people and new technologies have benefited people even with the most severe physical problems. It allows the disabled person to work, to maintain social contact, and to function independently in the community. It also encourages people to communicate and raises their self-esteem. Many cars, both big and small, come as standard, with automatic transmission, power assisted steering and with electric windows, and are more reliable and easier to drive these days.

Disabled people require information about their suitability to drive and the following questions may be addressed.
- Their safety to drive.
- The most suitable type of car to acquire.
- Any aids and adaptations that are required.
- Sources of finance, purchase, or hire of the vehicle.
- Insurance for driving and how to gain tax exemptions.
- How they can stow a wheelchair if one is used.
- How other people can be carried in the vehicle.
- How they can be assessed by an instructor with the necessary adaptations to a learner vehicle.
- Advice on alternative means of transportation if driving is not feasible.

The main medical barriers to driving are epilepsy, visual loss, cognitive deficits (in particular perceptual loss, memory loss, distraction and inattention, and intellectual loss), global dysphasia, severe mood changes, and blackouts, dizziness etc. Loss of vision and perception mean that driving would be very difficult and it is incumbent that the rehabilitation team assesses this before raising the expectations of a disabled person to return to driving. Epilepsy is a prescribed condition for driving, for which the Department of Transport has guidelines. The ban on driving has been shortened in recent years and 12 months of freedom of seizures while awake is the norm to allow a return of a driving licence. This applies to a single fit, as well as to post-traumatic epilepsy. Nocturnal epilepsy, when seizures occur during sleep, must not have been present for 3 years.

Vehicle modifications

Virtually anything, it seems nowadays, can be done to a vehicle to make it suitable for a disabled person to drive. However, transportation is not only about the disabled people getting behind the steering wheel. Access is also an issue. Vehicles can be adapted to allow transfer from a wheelchair to a car seat, or by build modification to allow the disabled person to travel in their own wheelchair in the vehicle. A whole host of seat cushions, steering aids, and hand-operated controls (brakes, accelerators, etc.) can be fitted in or after manufacture so that specific adaptations do not necessarily need to be made. Certain items are now indispensable, such as a car telephone, in order to summon help quickly, if required.

Many rehabilitation centres are able to assess people on their own premises, but the Forum of UK Mobility Centres see large numbers of people. Interestingly, many otherwise able-bodied people also undertake a disabled driving assessment on their 70th birthday in order to give them the confidence to continue driving beyond that age.

Chapter 13

Behavioural disorders

Background

Problems with behaviour are regrettably quite common in rehabilitation units, particularly those dealing with people with traumatic brain injury. The period of confusion during post-traumatic amnesia can often lead to inappropriate behaviour. Fortunately in most people behavioural problems are relatively mild and short-lived. It is only a minority who develop longer-term persistent and seriously disruptive behaviour. This group will often need specialist assistance from a neurobehavioural unit. However, the majority can, and should, be adequately managed in a rehabilitation unit. Almost all units, and particularly those catering for people with traumatic brain injury, should have access to a clinical neuropsychologist who is likely to be the leading figure in assessment and management of people with behavioural disorders.

Behavioural problems can follow any brain injury but are most common following traumatic brain injury. They are also particularly common after anoxic brain injury and less so after stroke or multiple sclerosis. It is also worth remembering that people with pre-existing behavioural problems secondary to mental illness or learning disabilities can also suffer traumatic brain injury and exhibit a worsening (or sometimes an improvement) of their previous difficulties.

Behavioural problems can be grouped into two broad categories: inappropriate excessive behaviour and inappropriate lack of behaviour. The former, which is the commoner form after traumatic brain injury, can present with a variety of difficulties:
• Verbal aggression.
• Physical aggression.
• Shouting at staff members or other clients.
• Aggressive refusal to cooperate with the rehabilitation programme.
• Inappropriate sexual behaviour.
• Impulsivity.
• Extreme egocentrism.

The most dramatic end of the behavioural spectrum is termed 'episodic dyscontrol syndrome'. In this syndrome the individual can have sudden aggressively violent outbursts with little or no warning.

At the other end of the spectrum inappropriate lack of behaviour can include:
• Apathy.
• Lack of initiation.
• Requirement for prompting and cajoling to undertake simple daily living tasks.

In these circumstances individuals are often labelled as lacking in motivation. Such a label should be avoided. The implication of lack of motivation or laziness is that it is the fault of the individual and therefore there is little that can be done to correct the problem. Such a label can produce a nihilistic approach to therapy which is in no one's interest.

Learning theory

Behavioural management techniques are normally based on various classical learning theories. Thus a brief overview of learning theory is desirable. This is a complex and specialist subject and this brief description will have to be simplistic. There are three broad areas of learning theory:

- Classical conditioning.
- Operant conditioning.
- Observational or vicarious conditioning.

Classical conditioning

This is classical Pavlovian theory and explains behaviour in terms of learning that two stimuli tend to go together. In his classic experiments Pavlov showed that a dog salivated on presentation of a stimulus such as a bell or light if, on previous occasions, this stimulus had been associated with the presentation of food. The bell or light is known as the *conditional stimulus* and the salivation as the *conditional response*. This association can be broken if one stimulus becomes unassociated with the other—known as extinction. Sometimes the association can also generalize with similar conditional stimuli, such as a different light or a different sound.

Operant conditioning

Operant or instrumental conditioning occurs when individuals correctly learn the association between some action of their own and an environmental consequence. This can include the delivery of food or giving praise. Procedures adapted from operant conditioning studies form the majority of behavioural modification techniques.

Classical and operant conditioning are both forms of associative learning. In other words the individual learns a linkage between one experience and another. There is now good evidence, particularly from animal studies, that shows that associative learning abilities are retained even in the presence of severe brain damage. Associative learning has even been demonstrated when people are still in coma. This is why associative learning techniques are the most successful in those with brain damage.

Observational or vicarious conditioning

This is learning that occurs through observation. A child, for example, can learn to be fearful of spiders if the parent is seen to be frightened. It is likely that such learning requires relatively intact cognitive processes. Cognitive approaches to retraining are usually more relevant when cognitive impairments are specific rather than more global.

Approaches to the management of behavioural problems—definition of the problem

There are two questions that need to be answered here:
- What is the problem?
- Who has the problem?

What is the problem?

The answers must be tightly defined. It is insufficient to say that X is aggressive. X may only be aggressive in particular circumstances or with particular people or doing particular things.

Who has the problem?

Sometimes the behavioural problem in the individual is relatively mild but has been overemphasized or exaggerated by carers, family, or staff. Sometimes staff could require the individual to be at a particular place at a particular time—say for medication or at mealtimes. If the individual is not in the right place at the right time then they may be labelled as having behavioural disorders whereas in fact they may not be hungry or not agree with the necessity of being at a particular place.

Once it is agreed by all concerned that there is a problem with a particular behaviour then it needs further analysis.

Approaches to the management of behavioural problems—study and analyse the problem

A useful approach is ABC—Antecedent, Behaviour, Consequence. In order to further analyse the problem individuals will need to be carefully observed. If resources permit then this is best done by a dedicated member of staff over a prolonged period of time. It is usually difficult, if not impossible, for an individual's behaviour to be properly studied and analysed on a busy rehabilitation ward without some dedicated staff time.

The *antecedent* behaviour determines what pre-dates or seems to trigger the inappropriate behaviour. Different questions to ask include:
• In what circumstances does it occur?
• What appears to trigger it?
• What appears not to trigger it?
• Is it situation specific?
• Is it environment specific?
• Is it person specific?
• Is there no pattern at all?

Next, the *behaviour* itself needs close analysis:
• What are the characteristics of the behaviour?
• What form does it take?
• How long does it last?
• To who is it directed?
• To what is it directed?
• How often does it occur?

Next, *consequence* (what are the consequences of the behaviour?):
• Is there an observed benefit?
• Does it lead to reward or another form of positive reinforcement?
• Does the individual calm down quickly or slowly?

After such a period of close observation a pattern usually emerges—it is unusual for behavioural disturbance not to be triggered by anything and to have no pattern at all.

Approaches to the management of behavioural problems—formulate the treatment plan

After definition and study of the problem it is usually possible to define a specific behaviour that is to be targeted. It is usually best to work on one or a very few behaviours at any one time. As with all rehabilitation processes a measuring instrument needs to be devised in order to monitor the defined goal. Intangible outcomes—such as X is less aggressive—are not adequate. Specific measures are required, such as how many times X is aggressive over a given period of time or at a particular time of the day. Specific goals will often require continued close observation, and this in turn often still requires a dedicated and trained member of staff to undertake observation.

Specific treatment methodologies

Increasing desirable behaviours

Desirable behaviours can be increased in a number of different ways. The commonest method is by positive reinforcement. A positive reinforcement is something which is delivered immediately following the occurrence of a positive behaviour which will increase the probability of that behaviour being repeated. Such reinforcement should be as close to the behaviour as possible. The reinforcement can be tangible, such as food and drink, less tangible, such as praise, or be a conditional reinforcer where the person must learn the relative value of the reinforcement by receiving, for example, tokens. The tokens can then be exchanged for later secondary reinforcers, such as coffee or snacks.

The reinforcement should be given immediately after the behaviour occurs and in a consistent and clear manner. All members of the rehabilitation unit must know the behavioural approaches being adopted so that every time a particular behaviour occurs it can be appropriately reinforced by the same means.

There are a number of other related techniques:
- *Shaping*—shaping involves reinforcement of the small steps towards an eventual desired behaviour. If, for example, someone refuses to dress in the mornings then they could be initially rewarded for just looking at their clothes, then perhaps touching the clothes or putting them in an appropriate place, and then rewarded step-by-step over a period of time for each item of clothing that is correctly put on. Eventually the small reinforcers are withdrawn and larger steps, such as dressing the top half of the body without prompts, are reinforced until finally positive reinforcement is only given after completion of the entire task.
- *Fading* can occur if prompting is required and after some time that level of prompt is withdrawn.
- *Modelling* is imitation of the desired behaviour by a member of staff and such imitation is slowly withdrawn. This observational conditioning will often require a higher degree of cognitive function than the simpler associative learning techniques.

- *Environmental restructuring*—this is sometimes needed in order to reduce the chances that a situation occurs in which the behaviour can be triggered. If, for example, someone easily gets angry if they cannot coordinate their cutlery and plate then use of non-slip mats, plate guards, and adapted cutlery could make eating easier and reduce inappropriate behaviours.

Decreasing undesirable behaviours

There are two basic methods to decrease undesirable behaviours:
- *Punishment* involves the presentation of an aversive stimulus or removal of a positive stimulus immediately following the inappropriate behaviour.
- *Extinction* occurs when the reinforcer is no longer delivered to a previously reinforced response.

There are various forms of punishment:
- *Time out on the spot* (TOOTS)—this involves denying attention to behaviours, such as screaming or complaining, by either, for example, continuing with a conversation as if oblivious to the behaviour or simply by walking away.
- *Situational time out*—this involves removal of the person either from the activity to another part of the room or to a separate room, without providing verbal reinforcement.
- *Seclusion time out*—this is where the individual is placed in a bare room for periods of about 5 minutes—there are now doubts about whether this can be ethically justified.
- *Response cost*—if a token economy is being used to reward someone after positive behaviour then the same tokens can be removed after inappropriate behaviour.

Overall these techniques do require a considerable amount of skill, planning, and staff time. The programme can take several weeks to have an effect and sometimes it can be very difficult to generalize behavioural improvements into a broader setting. Some authorities say that such behavioural management programmes cannot really be applied in a general rehabilitation or hospital environment. However, in non-specialist units small-scale specific behavioural alterations can be made, although staff time and resources can be a problem.

Drug therapy

Behavioural management programmes should not rely on the use of sedative, anxiolytic, or psychotropic medication. Indeed such drugs can often worsen behaviour. Occasionally the use of such a drug on a general medical ward where there is real risk to other staff or patients can be justified but, in general, drugs should be avoided in the management of any behavioural disorder. There are some exceptions; in the more severe explosive forms of behaviour—the episodic dyscontrol syndrome—then anti-convulsants can be helpful, including carbamazepine, gabapentin, and lamotrigine.

Some would use the serotoninergic antidepressant trazodone, whilst others would advocate the use of lithium or beta blockade with metoprolol. If severe agitation requires treatment then buspirone is useful. Individuals with inappropriate lack of behaviour can sometimes respond to central stimulants such as dexamphetamine or methylphenidate, but such medication should be used with caution.

The drug management of behavioural disturbances is a complicated field and needs specialist advice and management.

Approaches to the management of behavioural problems—evaluation

After an appropriate period of intervention the behavioural strategy will need evaluation and perhaps the strategy itself or the goals will need readjustment. Behavioural management is a dynamic phenomenon and specific goals and targets will need constant review. However, unlike some aspects of physical rehabilitation, behavioural rehabilitation can take many months. Severe behavioural problems can take a year or more to change and are sometimes very resistant to generalization into other settings. Fortunately many behaviours arising in the recovery phase of traumatic brain injury, particularly around the period of emergence from post-traumatic amnesia, are short-lived and generally responsive to behavioural manipulation.

Overall, behavioural disorders are quite common following brain injury and can be a significant source of disruption to the rehabilitation programme. However, in most people such behaviours are short-lived and can be relatively easily managed by a simple behavioural management approach. However, even simple behaviours can be time-consuming for staff and must be delivered in a consistent fashion by the whole unit as well as by carers and family. Despite the problems, behavioural intervention can produce gratifying improvements for many people and enable them to lead a more independent life where otherwise some form of restrictive environment may have been necessary.

Further reading

1. Tyerman A and King N (2008). *Psychological approaches to rehabilitation after traumatic brain injury*. Blackwell Publishing, Oxford.
2. Williams WH and Evans JJ (2003). *Biopsychosocial approaches in neurorehabilitation: assessment and management of neuropsychiatric, mood and behavioural disorders*. Taylor & Francis, Basingstoke.
3. Wilson B, Herbert C, and Shiel A (2003). *Behavioural approaches to neuropsychological rehabilitation: optimizing rehabilitation procedures*. Psychology Press, Hove.

Chapter 14

Psychiatric problems and rehabilitation

Background

People with physical disabilities are not immune to psychiatric problems and people with psychiatric problems are not immune to acquiring physical disability as a result of trauma or disease. People with some specific psychiatric problems such as personality disorders, substance abuse, and alcoholism are particularly prone to acquiring physical disability, secondary to risk-taking or risk-attracting behaviour. In addition, brain injury itself can be associated with specific psychiatric problems. There is still much debate about whether such difficulties as depression, anxiety, or more profound problems such as psychosis are secondary to intrinsic brain damage or simply a secondary result of a reaction to such damage. In the end the causation is of little consequence as individuals will still need appropriate psychiatric assistance. There is no evidence that a person, for example, with depression in the context of physical disability is any more or less likely to respond to appropriate treatment than someone with an endogenous or reactive depression.

Rehabilitation units should obviously have access to a skilled multidisciplinary psychiatric team, particularly for people with more profound or chronic psychiatric problems. The following sections do not attempt to be a substitute for a psychiatric textbook but the management of the commonest psychiatric problems should certainly be part of the armamentarium of the rehabilitation team. Many rehabilitation units use some form of screening questionnaire to detect psychiatric problems—particularly depression and anxiety. Regrettably many self-report mood scales include a variety of somatic symptoms, which in themselves can be part of the associated physical disability. Such symptoms might include insomnia, weight loss, anorexia, early morning waking, and loss of libido. Thus, it may be best to use mood scales that exclude such somatic symptoms. Two scales worth noting are:

- The Hospital Anxiety and Depression Scale.[1,2]
- The Wimbledon Self Report Scale.[3]

Both these scales exclude somatic items and are valid and reliable as screening measures for anxiety and depression. They both require self completion of a few simple questions about enjoyment, worry, lack of interest etc. They are both quick to administer. The *General Health Questionnaire* (GHQ 28) is also well developed as a screening measure for depression and anxiety but does include somatic and social dimensions.[4]

These scales should not be used as the only measures of assessment, but are useful screening tools; appropriate cut off points could be used for further referral to an appropriate psychiatric or psychological assessment.

The commonest psychiatric problems encountered in rehabilitation units include depression, anxiety, post-traumatic stress disorder, and emotional lability.

References

1. Zigmond A and Snaith P (1983). Hospital Anxiety and Depression Scale. *Acta Psychiatrica Scandinvacia*, **67**, 361–70.
2. ⫠ The Hospital Anxiety and Depression (HAD) Scale is available online at http://www. glassessment.co.uk
3. Coughlan A and Storey P (1988). The Wimbledon Self Report Scale: emotional mood appraisal. *Clinical Rehabilitation*, **2**, 207–13.
4. Goldberg DP and Hillier VF (1979). A scaled version of the General Health Questionnaire. *Psychological Medicine*, **9**, 139–45.

Depression

Depressive illness is remarkably common after acquired physical disability. It occurs in around 50% of people following stroke and severe head injury. It is even commoner at some point during progressive neurological disability, such as multiple sclerosis and motor neuron disease. People with congenital disabilities or childhood-acquired disabilities also have periods when they are particularly prone to depression. This is often true at times of life change, such as around puberty or when striving to be independent and leaving the parental home.

There is a continuum of depressive illness, from feeling temporarily low to sustained major depression with risk of suicide. The current accepted classification is usually based on the American Psychiatric Association criteria published as a *Diagnostic and Statistical Manual for Psychiatric Disorders* (*DSM IV*). However, such a formal diagnosis is probably not necessary in the setting of rehabilitation unit.

- Depression is usually characterized by:
  - Sustained unpleasant mood either described directly as depression or as sadness, unhappiness, or the inability to feel pleasure (anhedonia).
- Behavioural accompaniments:
  - Social withdrawal.
  - Physical slowing.
  - Crying.
- Cognitive accompaniments:
  - Ideas of hopelessness, worthlessness, and guilt.
- Physiological or biological accompaniments:
  - Anorexia.
  - Weight loss.
  - Insomnia.
  - Early morning waking.
  - Loss of libido.

Treatment of depression

There are various labels for the different forms of depression including *adjustment disorder* (temporarily linked to a stressor; tends to resolve over <6 months) or *major depression* (more severe and more persistent). However, the label is less important than the diagnosis and determination of whether it is actually contributing to an impairment of function. If depression is adversely affecting function in any way then treatment should be initiated. There are two broad approaches:

- Psychological strategies
- Psychotropic medication.

Psychological strategies

Psychological strategies depend primarily on an understanding and sympathetic relationship between the counsellor, psychologist or psychotherapist, and the person with depression. The following points are key to appropriate management:

- Information about and explanation of the nature of the depression.
- Detailed exploration of ideas and knowledge about the person's illness and their views on prognosis.
- A broad-ranging discussion on the overall impact of the physical illness and depressive illness on the family, social, and work relationships.
- Discussion to bring out potential stressors and triggers to day-to-day variations in mood.
- Development of coping strategies.

There are various specific counselling or psychotherapeutic approaches that have been used and published and it is not appropriate or possible in this section to go through these strategies. However, the following may be used:

- Cognitive behavioural therapy.
- Client-centred approach of Karl Rogers.
- Rational emotive therapy.
- Gestalt therapy.

There are other approaches that may:

- Improve motivation.
- Increase treatment adherence.
- Overcome apathy and inertia.

It is important to note that many anti-depressive cognitive strategies do require a reasonably intact cortex and may be inappropriate for those with more severe forms of brain damage. In such people some would advocate the use of medication.

Medication

Medication does have an important place in the management of acute affective disorders and in the prevention of recurrent problems. The following are frequently used:

- Lithium for bipolar disorders.
- Older tricyclic anti-depressants (amitriptyline, dosulepin, clomipramine, and imipramine): these are useful anti-depressants but usage is often limited by troublesome anti-cholinergic side-effects (urinary retention,

constipation, and dry mouth are of particular relevance in the physically disabled population) and sedative properties.
- Newer tetracyclic anti-depressants and 5HT uptake inhibitors, such as fluoxetine and fluvoxamine.
- Specialist use of other anti-depressant agents, such as monoamine-oxidase inhibitors or, for severe mood swings, anti-convulsants, such as carbamazepine.
- ECT in the most severe cases.

The latter categories should probably only be used by a formal psychiatric team.

Anti-depressant medication should be used for several months and most authorities would recommend continuation of medication for at least 6 months and probably longer in more severe cases.

There is little evidence that suggests that one particular antidepressant drug regimen is better than another; there has been a recent Cochrane review.[1] The authors in this study found no evidence to support the routine use of pharmacotherapeutic or psychotherapeutic treatment for depression after stroke but did find some evidence of an improvement on the depression rating scales, although in some cases with an increase in the proportion of participants with anxiety at the end of the follow-up period. Drug treatment for depression in the context of neurological disorders should really only be undertaken by experts in the field. The side effects of such medication in the context of brain damage can often outweigh the advantages of the treatment. The dosage of antidepressants used in these circumstances also needs careful adjustment although there is no evidence that depression in neurological disorder needs any different dosage regimen from antidepressant medication in mental health disorders.

References
1. Hackett ML, Anderson CS, and House AO (2004). Interventions for treating depression after stroke. *Cochrane Database of Systematic Reviews*, Issue 3, Article No. CD003437.

Anxiety

Anxiety, like depression, is a common companion to physical disability. Anxiety also has physiological, behavioural, and cognitive accompaniments. Symptoms can include:

- Feeling of fearful anticipation.
- Irritability.
- Restlessness.
- Worry.
- Poor concentration.
- Feeling of tightness in the chest or difficulty breathing.
- Cardiovascular symptoms, such as palpitations.
- Gastrointestinal symptoms, such as dry mouth, difficulty swallowing, loose bowel motions.
- Musculoskeletal problems, such as ache and tension in the scalp, neck, or shoulders.
- Sleep problems, such as difficulty getting to sleep and restless sleep.
- Appetite disturbance.
- Central nervous system problems, such as blurring of vision, paraesthesia, and dizziness.
- Avoidance of anxiety-provoking situations, such as agoraphobia.
- Avoidance of physical activity or even avoidance of human company.

The latter problems, in a rehabilitation setting, can be interpreted as anti-social behaviour or lack of initiative and drive which are simply secondary to the brain injury, whereas treatment of the anxiety state may produce benefit.

Treatment

Psychological problems and/or medication can be used and include:

- Specific anxiety management training programmes, including relaxation techniques and distraction techniques.
- Specific counselling techniques as listed in the section on depression above.
- Anxiolytic medication—this should be avoided if possible but benzodiazepines are relatively safe and effective anxiolytics. Treatment should, if at all possible, be short term. Withdrawal can be difficult with a risk of rebound anxiety.
- Anti-depressants will often have an anti-anxiety effect and can be used even in the absence of depression.

It is very important to stress that anxiety can be caused or certainly worsened by insufficient information and explanation about current or potential new symptoms or about the natural history or prognosis of the disorder. Effective and sympathetic communication is probably the best anxiolytic and thus appropriate prevention and management is the responsibility of the whole rehabilitation team.

Post-traumatic stress disorder (PTSD)

PTSD can occur after someone has been exposed to a traumatic event. The seriousness of the event is not necessarily a good guide to the severity of the symptoms as individuals will respond differently to the same stressors. Paradoxically the most severe brain injuries are usually associated with a period of post-traumatic amnesia and inability to recall the traumatic event and some authorities have said that post-traumatic stress disorder cannot, by definition, exist in such people. This is probably not true as individuals can develop symptoms after being told the details of the accident or trauma. There are specific diagnostic criteria published by the American Psychiatric Association (*Diagnostic and Statistical Manual of Mental Disorders (DSM IV)*).[1] Basically the diagnosis rests on:

• Persistent re-experience of the event.
• Recurrent or intrusive distressing recollections.
• Recurrent or intrusive distressing nightmares related to the event.
• Avoidance of the scene of the trauma.
• Intense distress secondary to various triggers that symbolize or resemble part of the event.

The latter will result in efforts to avoid thoughts or feelings about the trauma and feelings of detachment or estrangement from others.

There are often persistent symptoms of:

• Increased arousal.
• Difficulty falling asleep.
• Irritability.
• Problems with concentration.
• Exaggerated startle response.

In many people these symptoms are relatively minor and short-lived. However, in others the symptoms can be persistent and long term and have a major effect on lifestyle and quality of life.

In such people specific psychological referral should be made as a number of treatment strategies have been shown to be beneficial. Cognitive behavioural therapy, for example, is useful as are various forms of group therapy, and if the problem has a bearing on the whole family then couple therapy or family therapy can be helpful.

Medication should be avoided, but depression and anxiety symptoms, which may need medication, can co-exist.

A recent Cochrane review found that medication treatments can be effective in treating PTSD. The review supported the use of SSRIs as first-line agents in the pharmacotherapy of PTSD. There is also evidence that cognitive behavioural therapy can be effective as well as evidence of the efficacy of eye movement desensitization and reprocessing (EMDR) but this technique may be difficult in those with brain injury who may already have disturbed eye movement.[2,3]

References

1. ⚲ Available at http://psych.org/MainMenu/Research/DSMIV.aspx
2. Stein DJ, Ipser JC, and Seedat S (2000). Pharmacotherapy for post-traumatic stress disorder (PTSD). *Cochrane Database of Systematic Reviews*, Issue 4, Article No. CD002795.
3. Bisson J and Andrew M (2005). Psychological treatment of post-traumatic stress disorder (PTSD). *Cochrane Database of Systematic Reviews*, Issue 2, Article No. CD003388.

Emotionalism

A number of disorders affecting the brain can lead to disturbance of emotionality—disturbance of the normal control or expression of emotion. There are two syndromes:
- Pathological crying and laughing.
- Emotional lability.

Pathological crying and laughing
- This is provoked by non-emotional stimuli.
- There is no affect that accompanies the pathological laughing and crying.
- The emotional expression cannot be controlled and the emotional behaviour is stereotyped.

Emotional lability
- This is produced by emotionally appropriate stimuli and often will look like normal crying or laughing but the trigger for such lability appears to be set at a different level from the 'normal' population. However, the distinction between these two syndromes is blurred and many would now prefer the term emotionalism for both phenomena.
- The problem is probably a direct manifestation of brain pathology rather than indicating any underlying emotional disturbance. Obviously a diagnosis of co-existent depression, anxiety, or post-traumatic stress disorder can be very difficult in such circumstances. However, emotionalism does seem to respond quite well to small doses of anti-depressant medication. The response can be dramatic to doses that would not normally be expected to have an anti-depressive effect. Sometimes modest doses of anti-convulsant medication, particularly carbamazepine, can also be helpful.
- A recent Cochrane review confirmed the efficacy of antidepressant medication but also demonstrated a lack of reliable data.[1]

References

1. House AO, Hackett ML, Anderson CS *et al.* (2004). Pharmaceutical interventions for emotion-alism after stroke. *Cochrane Database of Systematic Reviews*, Issue 2, Article No. CD003690.

Further reading

1. Tyerman A and King N (2008). *Psychological approaches to rehabilitation after traumatic brain injury*. Blackwell Publishing, Oxford.

Chapter 15

Cognitive and intellectual function

Background and terminology

Cognition is the term that refers to all the processes involved in perceiving, learning, remembering, and thinking. Thus, cognitive problems are very common in any process that affects brain function. The key to helping people with cognitive problems is accurate assessment of the nature of the problem. This should be followed by clear-cut information and advice about the nature of the problem—both to the affected person and the family. Until recent years neurologists and neuropsychologists had to stop at this point as there was little functional assistance that could be offered. This is now less true, and there are a number of useful strategies designed to improve various cognitive problems or at least to help the individual cope with them better. Cognitive rehabilitation is a relatively new and largely untested field but rapid progress is being made.

The terminology used in cognitive assessment can be confusing and the following two sections offer a very simple guide to cognitive terminology.

Perceptual problems

Perception is the cognitive process that enables us to make sense of our environment. This can be through any of the senses but the most important are:

- *Sight*—visual perception.
- *Hearing*—auditory perception.
- *Touch*—tactile perception.

Perceptual deficits of taste and smell do exist but in humans are of less functional significance. Perception can be affected in a number of ways.

Agnosia

Agnosia is the inability to perceive that cannot be explained by a primary sensory disorder or a deficit of naming or severe general intellectual impairment. Each of the senses has a specific agnosia. Visual agnosia is the most important.

Thus, *visual agnosia* is the inability to recognize objects which cannot be explained on the basis of a primary sight disorder or on the basis of a language problem or general intellectual loss. There are more precise visual agnostic syndromes including:

- *Colour agnosia*—loss of the ability to recognize colours.
- *Prosopagnosia*—loss of the ability to recognize familiar faces.
- *Simultanagnosia*—loss of the ability to perceive all the elements of a scene simultaneously and interpret that scene, i.e. recognition of parts of the scene but not the whole.

The other senses also have their own forms of agnosia, such as tactile agnosia and auditory agnosia.

Neglect

Neglect is the failure to attend to one side of a space or one side of self by the relevant sense. Individuals with *visual neglect*, for example, will commonly bump into things on the affected side or fail to see food on one side of the plate thinking they have finished the meal when in fact it has only been half eaten. This is commonly, but not always, a right-hemisphere problem and is particularly common after stroke.

Apraxias

These are perceptual problems in which a person without general intellectual decline and without weakness, ataxia, motor, or sensory deficit is unable to execute previously learnt skills or gestures. The apraxias can be subdivided into:

- *Ideational apraxia*—where there is a complete failure to conceive or formulate an action either spontaneously and/or to a command.
- *Ideomotor apraxia*—where the individual knows and remembers the plan of action but simply cannot carry it out.

There can be quite specific forms of apraxia including:
- *Constructional apraxia*—refers to problems in putting things together in two or three dimensions, such as jigsaw puzzles.
- *Dressing apraxia*—the inability to dress properly and remember the right clothing in the right sequence. This is common after stroke and can lead to people being completely unable to dress or, in less serious cases, simply trying to put their trousers on the wrong way around or putting underpants on after the trousers.

Language and communication problems

These are discussed in Chapter 10, but language problems are a common accompaniment to other cognitive difficulties.

Dysphasia

Dysphasia is a generic term for the understanding of language. It is usually divided into non-fluent and fluent aphasias:

- **Non-fluent aphasia** usually corresponds to damage to the anterior part of the brain. As a generalization people with such aphasias have great difficulty in expressing themselves with the correct words in the right sequence. Part of the non-fluent aphasic syndrome used to be known as Broca's aphasia. There are now recognized to be three basic non-fluent aphasias—*Broca's aphasia, transcortical motor aphasia,* and *global aphasia.* The distinction between these aphasias is outside the scope of this volume.
- **Fluent aphasias** tend to result from damage to the posterior part of the brain and tend to lead to problems of understanding or comprehension. These used to be called receptive dysphasias and a well-known variety is Wernicke's aphasia. Once again there are now recognized to be three forms of fluent aphasia—*Wernicke's aphasia, transcortical sensory aphasia,* and *conduction aphasia.*

The subtleties of the classification are certainly important in making a formal functional assessment and are becoming important in terms of remediation of various communication problems. These difficulties are in the realm of the specialist speech and language therapist.

The various dysphasias do need to be distinguished from *dysarthria,* which is a problem of speech production usually due to brainstem or local mouth or pharyngeal pathology. Classically the individual has a slurring of speech, and once again there are various defined subtypes.

There is other language terminology:

- *Anomia*—specific naming ability causing problems naming particular objects.
- *Paraphasia*—production of an unintended or nonsense word (neologism).
- *Agrammaticism*—difficulty with grammar or structure of language.
- Various disorders causing problems with repetition.
- Problems repeating phrases.
- Often people with problems of language processing have related difficulties with reading (*dyslexia*), writing (*dysgraphia*), and calculating (*dyscalculia*).

Memory problems

Memory problems are probably the commonest cognitive problem following brain injury and the one that has the most profound impact on daily function. There has recently been much progress in the understanding of memory and some progress (☐ see Cognitive rehabilitation, p.226) in rehabilitation of memory difficulties. There are a number of dimensions of memory.

Different time spans

* *Immediate or working memory*—this is memory just for the previous few seconds, such as is required to hold a telephone number in the head whilst dialling. There are different forms of working memory according to the different senses used—*phrenological system* for auditory information, *visuo-spatial system* for visual information as well as a controlling *central executive system*.
* *Long-term memory*:
  * *Delayed*—memory for events that happened in the previous few minutes.
  * *Recent*—memory for events that happened in the previous days or weeks.
  * *Remote*—memory for events that happened several weeks to several years previously.
* *Prospective memory*—memory for things that need to be done in the future.

Different types of information

* *Semantic memory*—memory for factual knowledge.
* *Episodic memory*—memory for events and autobiographical material.
* *Procedural memory*—memory for skills and practical procedures; this is often preserved in brain injury when episodic and semantic memory is not.

Memory in different forms

* *Verbal memory*—memory for information in the form of words, both written and spoken.
* *Visual memory*—memory for things that have to be remembered in visual format.

Stages of remembering

All these different forms of memory need to go through different stages of encoding, storage, and later retrieval. Problems can arise at any of these stages for any of the different memories and thus one can see the complexity of trying to unravel the different forms of memory disorder.

Perhaps an example is useful. Remembering how to drive a car is a skill that will require procedural memory. The fact that a car is used to drive one to work is semantic memory and the fact that the car was actually used to drive to work that morning needs episodic memory. Memory that the car is made of metal and the tyres of rubber is semantic memory. There may be other memories about different cars that one has purchased in the past or particularly pleasant or unpleasant memories about particular cars.

A few other memory terms need to be described:
- *Retrograde amnesia* is usually associated with cerebral injury and applies to loss of memory prior to the injury, which is usually a very short period of time and normally only a few minutes.
- *Anterograde amnesia* applies to on-going memory disturbance after a particular trauma. The commonest form is *post-traumatic amnesia* (PTA), which describes the period of time after a cerebral insult before continuous day-to-day memory returns. The length of PTA is a good determinant of the severity of the injury and the prognosis for later recovery.

Memory is undoubtedly complicated and Fig. 15.1 illustrates a simple schematic summarizing, probably in an over-simplistic form, the different forms of memory.

Psychologists now have a number of standardized tests for assessment of the different forms of memory and a clinical neuropsychologist should be involved in the assessment and treatment of anyone with a memory problem, or indeed other cognitive problems.

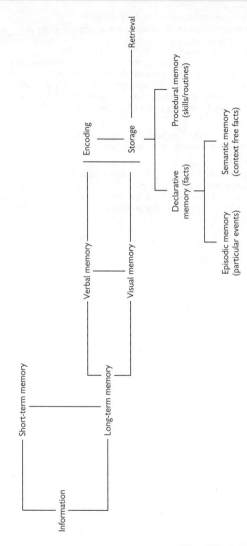

Fig. 15.1 Long-and short-term memory

Attention deficits and other problems of higher executive function

Attention is the ability to remain aware of one's surroundings. It is also the ability to selectively attend to important signals. One may be listening, for example, to music and can divert attention if someone starts a conversation even though the music is still playing. Problems with attention can easily result in difficulties with daily living. People with brain injuries have problems with *selective attention* and find it difficult to exclude less important inputs—the so-called cocktail party syndrome. At a party, for example, they may not be able to selectively attend to the person with whom they are talking if there are other background conversations or music. They may also have problems *alternating attention* from one task to another, such as when driving a car. They may have problems with *dividing attention* in order to respond simultaneously to two or more things at once, such as carrying on a conversation whilst driving.

There is also a cluster of symptoms that people classically show following damage to the frontal lobe brain structures. People with such damage often experience a large range of difficulties in everyday life. These symptoms used to be called the 'frontal lobe syndrome'. However, this label is rather unsatisfactory and implies a clear-cut syndrome. It is more helpful to categorize the particular problems in an individual person and the whole collection of symptoms is now known as the 'dysexecutive syndrome'. There are a number of characteristics which can be listed:

- Problems with abstract thinking.
- Impulsivity.
- Confabulation.
- Problems with planning.
- Euphoria.
- Temporal sequencing problems.
- Lack of insight and social awareness.
- Apathy and lack of drive.
- Disinhibition.
- Disturbed impulse control.
- Shallow affective responses.
- Aggression.
- Lack of concern.
- Perseveration (difficulty changing mindset).
- Restlessness.
- Inability to inhibit responses.
- Distractibility.
- Loss of decision-making ability.
- Lack of concern for social rules.

A look down this list will indicate the very wide variety of problems that can occur in the dysexecutive syndrome and the difficulties that can result in terms of everyday life and social functioning.

Cognitive rehabilitation

Is it possible to restore cognitive function? This has been a controversial question for a number of years and there is still limited evidence to make a definitive answer. Placebo-controlled, double-blind studies are very difficult, and some would say impossible, in this field and scientific progress has usually relied on single-case methodology. There is now some evidence that a number of cognitive problems are amenable to a rehabilitation strategy, including:

• Attention deficits.
• Unilateral neglect.
• Some deficits in communication, including dyslexia.
• Some aspects of memory dysfunction.

In broad terms functional benefit can derive from a broad cognitive approach that adopts two strategies:

• Bypass the problem or find another way to achieve the same goal.
• Use residual skills more effectively.

Finding a way around the problem

A number of strategies can be designed according to the individual problems. People can be provided with assistive equipment; individuals with memory problems, for example, can be taught to use external memory aids, such as diaries, lists, alarm clocks, timers, and tape recorders. Reminders on mobile phones are also useful. However, these methods are not always successful as people need some residual memory in order to remember what they are being reminded about! There are commercial systems that are radio-controlled and a central switchboard will transmit a message into a small communicator reminding the person what needs doing at that particular moment.

Another strategy is to rearrange the immediate environment in order to reduce cognitive input. Sometimes this will involve a rigid organization of daily life so that limited planning and organizational skills are required. A very structured day, with diaries and prompts from another party, can often assist someone with aspects of the dysexecutive syndrome. Organization of physical space, such as labelling drawers, doors, and kitchen utensils can be helpful. Sometimes simple measures can help such as supplying simple clothing with labels and Velcro® fastening for people with dressing apraxia. There are a whole variety of strategies that first need an accurate neuropsychological assessment and then application of a common-sense way to get around the problem.

Using residual skills more effectively

There are a number of techniques in this area that have mainly been developed in the field of memory. Mnemonic strategies have been used including *imagery*, where information is remembered by an association with a particular image. An example is the *PQRST* mnemonic. In this technique individuals are taught to Preview information, set Questions to themselves on the information, Read information over, State the information again, and Test the results. It is hoped by this method that the information is more deeply encoded. There are many other techniques that can use acronyms, rhymes, and systematic cueing, where a well-known series, such as the alphabet, is scanned through to cue an appropriate memory.

This, and many other techniques, are designed to use residual skills more efficiently and now have been shown to produce real functional benefit and lessen disability in many people. In an individual case a number of different strategies can be used. It is vital that the main carers and family are involved in the regular and routine implementation of an appropriate strategy.

Further reading

1. Baddeley AD, Kopelman M, and Wilson BA (2004). *The Essential Handbook of Memory Disorders for Clinicians*. John Wiley, Chichester.
2. Tulving E and Craik FIM (2000). *The Oxford Handbook of Memory*. Oxford University Press, Oxford.
3. Halligan PW, Kischka U, and Marshall JC (2003). *Handbook of Clinical Neuropsychology*. Oxford University Press, Oxford.
4. ⌂ www.cognitive-rehab.org.uk—website for the Society of Cognitive Rehabilitation which contains sub-pages on recommendations for best practice in cognitive rehabilitation therapy in the context of acquired brain injury.

Participation issues in rehabilitation

Introduction

Participation issues are concerned with the factors that affect the lives of people with disabilities. Although often outside the control of health professionals—as they are based on societal attitudes and governmental legislative policy—the rehabilitation team needs to develop links with professionals in employment, social services, and housing departments. Although this chapter has a UK orientation, the same principles apply in other societies. The details may change, but it is important to address participation and how societal barriers can be broken down to allow people with disabilities to play their full part in society. This chapter highlights the areas to be covered, but also the areas where most of the barriers exist. Society's attitude to people with disability is changing for the better, but there is a long way to go before disability discrimination ceases.

Finance and benefits

Problems faced

Low income

One of the greatest barriers to participation for disabled people is the lack of finance and financial control. Although paid employment is a valid goal for many younger people, the prospect of a return to work for many middle aged and older people will not be realistic because of their functional restriction or societal barriers and prejudices. Many disabled people have a low income from being unemployed, having to work part-time, or working in menial or low-paid jobs.

Increased expenditure

Equipment, increased clothing needs and heating costs, contributions to housing adaptations, travel, etc. are all present extra financial burden on people with disabilities, which go unrecognized by the majority of the population.

The benefits structure is very complicated and many people do not know to what they are entitled. Help is at hand in most towns and cities through Citizens Advice Bureaux and information desks of disabled people's organizations. Rehabilitation teams should have a working knowledge of people's rights on welfare and should know the appropriate information sources in their community. Table 16.1 gives a summary of some of the benefits.

Table 16.1 Summary of UK benefits

Situation	Benefit available
Incapable of work: previously employed	Statutory Sick Pay for 28 weeks
	Incapacity Benefit >28 weeks
Eligible for Incapacity Benefit (IB):	
Short-term sick for 28–52 weeks	Short-Term IB
Long-term sick for >52 weeks ± receiving high rate of DLA care component	Long-Term IB
IB started before age of 45 years	Incapacity Age Addition
Incapable of work: ≥16 hours work/week for ≥4 weeks, ≥16 years of age with disability or aged ≥25 years and usually working for ≥30 hours/week	Disabled Person's Working Tax Credit
Incapable of work: ≥16 hours work/week for ≥4 weeks, ≥16 years of age with disability or aged ≥25 years and usually working for ≥30 hours/week and looking after child dependants	Child Tax Credit
<60 years. Incapable of work: Insufficient to live on. Mean tested. Minimum income guaranteed.	Income Support
Unemployed	Income Support/Jobseekers' Allowance
Incapable of full-time work, but working <16 hours per week	Jobseekers' Allowance
Incapable of work from industrial injury or work-related illness	Industrial Injuries Disablement Benefit
War disablement	War disablement pension / War widows' pension
Disabled person aged <65 years requiring help with	Disability Living Allowance (DLA)
Personal care	Care component—low, middle, and high rates
Mobility	Mobility component—low & high rates
	'Motability' loan for vehicular transport
	Blue Badge' parking from Local Authority
	Road tax exemption
Disabled person aged ≥65 years requiring help with personal care	Attendance allowance
Injury due to violent crime	Criminal Injuries compensation
Vaccine damage	Vaccine damage payment
Help with living at home and requiring home improvements while on income support.	Housing Benefit, Council Tax Benefit
Other	Bus/Rail Pass for all aged ≥60 years

Education and further education

Children with disabilities have to remain in education until the age of 16 years in the UK, but further education facilities are available to the age of 19 years. The policy has been for many years to educate disabled children as far as possible in main-stream schools, but some have such significant needs, that special facilities are provided. See Tables 16.2 and 16.3.

'Statementing'

An assessment of a child's educational requirements. This is started at any time during a child's schooling and is formally reviewed in Years 8, 9, 10 and 11 to prepare both the child and the services for action to accommodate the transition to post-school life, whether that is in further education or not. It is a multidisciplinary process and contributions are made by GPs, therapists, nursing staff, social services, teachers, and educational psychologists. The parents have to agree it. As it is reviewed annually, it forms part of a rehabilitation framework for the young person at school, but service inadequacies exist.

Table 16.2 Legislation to date

Legislation	Date	Action/recommendation
Warnock Report	1978	Critical of state provision and identifying some of the educational special needs
Education Act	1981	Established a statement of children's educational needs. "Statementing"
Disabled Persons Act, Sections 5 & 6	1986	Important legislation. Identified young people's rights
Education Act	1993	Details of procedures and appeals
Education Act	1996	Refinement of above
National Service Framework for Elderly	2001	Defined NHS responsibilities for the management and rehabilitation of elderly people, including those who have suffered a stroke
National Service Framework for Long Term Conditions	2005	Highlights the impact of long-term conditions on healthcare in the UK. Defines 11 quality requirements to transform the way health and social care services support people with long-term neurologial conditions to live as independently as possible. Although the NSF focusses on people with long-term neurological conditions, much of the guidance it offers can apply to anyone living with a long-term condition

Table 16.3 Some comparisons of mainstream versus special schools

Advantages	Disadvantages
Larger schools likely to have better educational facilities	Bigger distances for the disabled child to cover. Increased energy consumption to get around may negate some educational advantages
Likely to have or aspire to higher educational achievement	Disabled child may feel alone in company of able-bodied children in large school
Mixing and competing with the general population	Less understanding of individual child's overall needs, particularly in time to achieve targets. Child may be seen as a poor achiever
Wider circle of friends	Lack of specialist teachers and specialist aids to teaching
School likely to be nearer than special school	Lack of on-site therapy facilities or therapists
Disability less likely to 'handicap' a child's ability to get on after school	Some facilities may be inaccessible

Employment

Disabled people in general have high unemployment rates, but only those with cognitive or severe physical problems are incapable of work. Several factors are important, not least the unwillingness (for a number of reasons) of employers wishing to take them on. The cost of lost employment to the nation is enormous and includes direct costs, lost productivity, and reduced services. The longer one is off work, the lower the chance of returning. This falls to ~50%, after 6 months of back pain, to 25% at 1 year and to 10% at 2 years. The commonest medical causes are musculoskeletal, mental health, and circulatory disorders.

Musculoskeletal'

- 1.78 million workers reporting sick (28% of those on benefits):
  - Back pain—642 000.
  - Neck/upper limb—512 000.
  - Lower limbs—212 000.
  - >1 site—178 000.
- Low back pain:
  - Highest incidence in agriculture, construction, food, nursing, retail industries.
  - 90 million working days lost through spinal disorders (£5–10 billion)

Mental health disorders

Account for 20% of sickness benefits payments—the highest cause in London. Most are minor problems rather than major psychiatric disease. Many are put down to pressures in the workplace (stress) and may be a reason for this being the second highest cause of health related premature retirement.

Circulatory disorders

Account for 13% of sickness benefits payments.

References

1. National service framework for long-term conditions (2005). HMSO, London.

Vocational rehabilitation

Definition

Vocational rehabilitation (VR)—the concept of enabling temporarily or permanently disabled individuals to access, return or remain in employment.[1] See Fig. 16.1.

VR schemes have the potential to give a 2–10 × return on costs through:
- Reduced sickness absence.
- Reduced early retirement.
- Increased productivity.
- Continued payment of taxes.
- Reduced payment of state benefits.

Team roles
- Rehabilitation physician:
  - Medical and disability assessment.
  - Prognostication.
  - Medical interventions.
  - Health service planning initiatives and development.
- Occupational therapists:
  - Traditional role in returning people to work.
  - Well placed to take up this role again (Fig. 16.2).
- Physotherapist:
  - Functional capacity assessment.
  - Manual handling education.
  - Pre-employment screening.
  - Post injury therapy.
  - Risk assessment between workers and work activities work hardening and work conditioning.
  - Workforce health promotion.
- Psychology:
  - Emotional and psychological assessments.
  - Treatments, e.g. cognitive behavioural therapy.

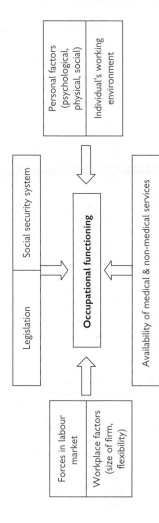

Fig. 16.1 Schematic view of VR

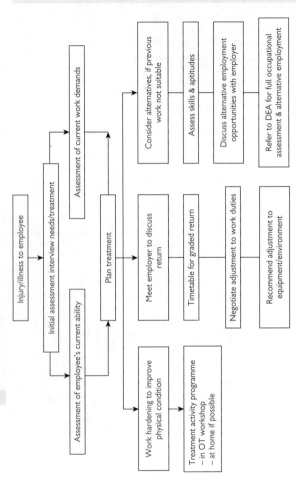

Fig. 16.2 Occupational therapy VR scheme

References

1. British Society of Rehabilitation Medicine (2000). *Vocational rehabilitation–the way forward*. Report of a working party. BSRM, London.

Transition to adult life—the disabled school leaver

The problem

Moving from the relatively well-coordinated facilities of school life to a less-structured adult environment can be a major change for people with disabilities and their families (Tables 16.4, 16.5, and Box 16.1). It is a time of great change for us all and young people with disabilities are less equipped to deal with it. On top of this there are organizational changes and the professional teams that the person and the family were so used to disappear. Paediatricians cease to provide services and their philosophy of total health care (where children are under the same specialist for acute and on-going health problems) is now replaced by a more fragmented service, where the person and family do not usually get to know their doctor/therapists as well. Disability tends to be higher among ethnic groups for whom there are already disadvantages and a greater burden.

Table 16.4 Additional legislation to consider

Legislation	Date	Action/recommendation
Disabled Persons Act Sections 5 & 6	1986	Important legislation. Identified the rights of young people
Children's Act	1989	Social Services' responsibilities change to adult provision at 19 years
Education Act	1996	Refinement of above
Disability Discrimination Act	1995	Enshrines some disabled person's rights

Table 16.5 Constraints for disabled young adults

Constraint	Examples
Resources	Lack of appropriate facilities
Personal ability	Low self-esteem and self-image
Family concern	Decreased aspirations for child and letting go of childhood
Service mismatching	Failure to match client with facility

Box 16.1 Highlight of mismatch of service provision and individual needs

- Lack of coordinated rehabilitation service.
- Shortage of skilled specialists in health and social services.
- Poor liaison between services, fragmenting response to individuals.
- Lack of accessible and up-to-date information resource for service users and for providers.
- Inadequate provision of certain services.
- Inadequate provision of and lack of choice of residential accommodation.
- Inadequate day care provision outside city centres.

Epidemiology (Table 16.6)

Table 16.6 Incidence and prevalence of some diseases in young adults

Disease/injury	Incidence per 10^6	Prevalence per 10^6	Prevalence trend
Congenital:			
Cerebral palsy	200	–	Static
Spina bifida	Variable	2	Down
Muscular dystrophy—all types	1–3/8000 live births	90	Down
Neurological rarities	Make large group together	–	Down
Cystic fibrosis	40/2500 live births	–	Up in >15-year-olds
Acquired:			
Head injury	300	150	Up
Spinal injury	10–15	–	Static
Juvenile chronic arthritis	16	<113	Static
Multiple sclerosis	48	99–198	Static

Requisite skills for a young adult (Table 16.7)

Table 16.7 Additional legislation to consider

Maintenance skills			Life skills				
Health	Self-care	Domestic	Mobility	Relationships	Leisure	Work	Self-development
• Nutrition • Exercise • Disease management • Disability management • Use of NHS resources (eg. GP, dentist)	• Feeding • Dressing • Hygiene	• Food collection, preparation, storage • Clothes maintenance • Home cleaning/ maintenance • Home safety • Money management	• Indoors • Threshold • Outdoors • On foot, in wheelchair, using public and private transport	• Sexual • Family • Social • Work • Community • Other	• Hobbies • Sport	• Direct work skills and mobility to and within workplace • Posture and seating	• Assertiveness • Negotiation • Time management • Money management • Information acquisition & use • Career development

Service provision

Dedicated teams have an advantage over an ad hoc approach to service delivery through giving disabled young people better knowledge, information and therefore access to services (Fig. 16.3). They aim to allow the establishment of an adult lifestyle and improve the quality of life of young people with physical disabilities aged between 16 and 25–30 years of age through:

- Health care and personal issues—disability, psychosexual, genetic counselling (NHS).
- Equipment for daily living, education and employment (NHS/SSD/D of Schools, DWP).
- Information (all).
- Independent living skills (NHS/ D of Schools).
- Social needs, personal care, finance and occupational activity (NHS, SSD, DWP).
- Further education and training (D of Schools).
- Transport, mobility and access (all, NHS).
- Housing (LA).
- Leisure and recreation facilities (SSD/NHS).

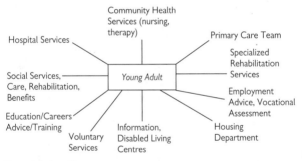

Fig. 16.3 Links with services

Multiple sclerosis

Background

Multiple sclerosis (MS) is the commonest cause of severe physical disability in young adults. The progressive and changing nature of the condition combined with the complexity of the resulting disability makes MS one of the most serious challenges to the neurological rehabilitation team. These sections concentrate on the management of disability. Some background details are relevant and are described in the next few sections—epidemiology, natural history, and diagnosis.

Epidemiology

There is a well-known geographical variation in prevalence of MS. There is a strong trend for prevalence to increase with increasing latitude both north and south of the equator. This trend is even noticeable in the UK with lower prevalence rates in the southern part of the country compared with high prevalence rates in the northern Scottish islands—up to 258 per 100 000 population. The overall prevalence rate in the UK is around 120 per 100 000 population. Thus, in the UK a typical general practice with a population of around 2000 will have 2–3 people with MS on their list.

Incidence in the UK is around 2–6 per 100 000 per annum. In the context of this section it is more relevant to know the proportion of people with MS who are significantly disabled. Around two-thirds of the total MS population is thought to be moderately or severely disabled at any one time. About 80% of people are significantly disabled by 20 years post diagnosis. As the mean age of onset of MS is around 30 it follows that the burden of disability and handicap will fall in the 4th and 5th decades of life.

Natural history and prediction of prognosis

Life expectancy is only modestly shortened in MS. The median survival time is >40 years and as the average age of onset is in the 30s it can be seen there is only a small reduction of life expectancy. There are a few people with rapidly progressive MS who regrettably die within a few years of onset, but such a pattern is unusual. There are a number of different patterns of MS and a few salient points are as follows:

- Relapsing/remitting MS—periods of good health or remission followed by sudden symptoms or relapses—80% of people at onset.
- Secondary progressive MS—follows on from relapsing/remitting. There are gradually more or worsening symptoms with fewer remissions—50% of people with relapsing/remitting develop secondary progressive during the first 10 years of their illness.
- Primary progressive MS—from the beginning, symptoms gradually develop and worsen over time—10–15% of people at onset.
- Most will eventually convert to a progressive course—around 40% by 10 years; 60% by 15 years; and 70% by 25 years.
- The time to conversion to a progressive course is a good predictor of eventual disability—those who become progressive in a short period are more likely to have aggressive disease.
- Around 10% of the MS population do not ever convert to a progressive disease but continue to have relapsing/remitting disease and a benign course.
- It is difficult to predict progression of the disorder. However, the following are generally poor prognostic indicators:
  - Cerebellar symptoms and signs.
  - Polysymptomatic onset.
  - Increasing age of onset—particularly age of onset after 40 years.
  - Onset event giving a disability of greater than 3 on the Kurtzke Expanded Disability Status Scale (EDSS 📖 see Table 17.1, p.259).
  - Shorter intervals between relapses, particularly <1 year.
- Good prognostic signs are:
  - Monosymptomatic onset.
  - Early visual and sensory symptoms.
  - Absence of pyramidal signs 5 years after onset.
  - Absence of cerebellar signs 5 years after onset.
  - Younger age of onset.
  - Initial remitting course.

In the future more accurate prognosis may be possible with more widespread use of serial MRI scanning or by the monitoring of immune markers.

Diagnosis

Diagnosis of MS still rests largely on the traditional clinical skills of history and examination in an attempt to identify clinical lesions of the central nervous system at two or more different anatomical sites that have occurred on at least two separate occasions. Diagnosis is usually assisted or confirmed by:

- Examination of cerebrospinal fluid with evidence of oligoclonal banding and increase in immunoglobulin G production.
- Evoked potential examination.
- Neuroimaging, particularly MRI scanning.

When the history, examination, and investigations are combined MS can be diagnosed with reasonable certainty in the quite early stages. Studies show that the overwhelming majority of people wish to be told the diagnosis at the earliest possible opportunity. This phase of care is still poorly managed and a recent study showed that 10% of people still learnt of their diagnosis by accident or by an incautious remark:

- The diagnosis should be discussed in an unhurried atmosphere, allowing plenty of time for the individual and their family to discuss and ask questions.
- The individual should be given the opportunity for a second appointment soon after the first appointment when further questions have materialized.
- If they wish the individual should be given lay literature regarding MS. There is some particularly good literature produced by the MS Trust[1] and the MS Society[2] in the UK.
- The individual should be put in touch with the local support group who can act in a supportive and counselling role at a time of significant stress and anxiety.

References

1. ⚓ http://www.mstrust.org.uk/—website of the Multiple Sclerosis Trust in the UK
2. ⚓ http://www.mssociety.org.uk/—website of the Multiple Sclerosis Society in the UK

Precipitating and aggravating factors

Pregnancy

The 9 months of pregnancy are a fairly safe time with regard to MS relapse. However, there is a significant increase in relapse rate during the 3–6 months after the birth. Overall pregnancy, or the number of pregnancies, has no effect on subsequent disability. There is also no evidence that the contraceptive pill has any significant influence on the course of the disease.

Stress and life events

There are a number of anecdotal reports of a relationship between emotional shock and onset of the disease. However, more recent work has thrown some doubt on this relationship. Nevertheless, it is still generally accepted that 'extreme' life events, such as a major car accident or divorce, can precipitate a relapse. It is probable that the 'quality' rather than the 'quantity' of stressful life events appears to be the determinant of relapse risk. Obviously the closer the relapse to the stressful event then the more likely is the relationship.

Infection, immunization, and temperature

It is likely that systemic infection can precipitate a relapse but there is little evidence that it can precipitate the onset of MS. It is known that increase of body temperature, such as in a hot bath or after exertion, can be associated with a temporary worsening of symptoms (Uhthoff's phenomenon). There is, other than a few anecdotal reports, little evidence that immunization has any effect on the course of the disease.

Trauma and surgery

The evidence for trauma or surgery having any effect on MS is anecdotal, although there are a few apparently clear-cut cases showing such a relationship. Overall it is generally agreed that:
- There should be a close temporal relationship between the trauma and onset or exacerbation of MS, certainly within 3 months.
- The trauma should actually involve the central nervous system (e.g. brain injury after a road traffic accident).
- Preferably there should be a close anatomical relationship between the presumed site of the MS lesion and the anatomical site of the trauma.

Rating scales

As in all rehabilitation processes it is important for rehabilitation goals to be properly documented. It is probably more valuable to use a particular scale for the symptom that is being treated rather than use an overall disability scale. However, in the MS literature the Kurtzke Expanded Disability Status Scale (EDSS) is very widely used. There are problems with the scale, which mixes impairment with disability, but it is so widely used that it is reproduced in Table 17.1. It is often used in conjunction with a more detailed functional systems scoring, also developed by Kurtzke, but there are other disability scales available (📖 see Chapter 5).

Table 17.1 Kurtzke Expanded Disability Status Scale (EDSS)

Step	Description
0	Normal neurological exam (all grade 0 in functional systems (FS); cerebral grade 1 acceptable)
1.0	No disability, minimal signs in one FS (i.e. grade 1 excluding cerebral grade 1)
1.5	No disability, minimal signs in >one FS (more than one grade 1 excluding cerebral grade 1)
2.0	Minimal disability in one FS (one FS grade 2, others 0 or 1)
2.5	Minimal disability in two FS (two FS grade 2, others 0 or 1)
3.0	Moderate disability in one FS (one FS grade 3, others 0 or 1), or mild disability in three or four FS (three/four FS grade 2, others 0 or 1) though fully ambulatory
3.5	Fully ambulatory but with moderate disability in one FS (one grade 3) and one or two FS grade 2; or two FS grade 3; or five FS grade 2 (others 0 or 1)
4.0	Fully ambulatory without aid, self-sufficient, up and about some 12 hours a day despite relatively severe disability consisting of one FS grade 4 (others 0 or 1), or combinations of lesser grade exceeding limits of previous steps. Able to walk without aid or rest some 500 metres
4.5	Fully ambulatory without aid, up and about much of the day, able to work a full day, may otherwise have some limitation of full activity or require minimal assistance; characterized by relatively severe disability, usually consisting of one FS grade 4 (others 0 or 1) or combinations of lesser grades exceeding limits of previous steps. Able to walk without aid or rest for some 300 metres
5.0	Ambulatory without aid or rest for about 200 metres; disability severe enough to impair full daily activities (for example, to work a full day without special provisions). (Usual FS equivalents are one grade 5 alone, others 0 or 1; or combinations of lesser grades usually exceeding specifications for step 4.0.)
5.5	Ambulatory without aid or rest for about 100 m; disability severe enough to preclude full daily activities. (Usual FS equivalents are one grade 5 alone, others 0 or 1; or combinations of lesser grades usually exceeding specifications for step 4.0.)
6.0	Intermittent or unilateral constant assistance (cane, crutch, or brace) required to walk about 100 metres with or without resting. (Usual FS equivalents are combinations with more than two FS grade 3+.)
6.5	Constant bilateral assistance (canes, crutches, or braces) required to walk about 20 metres without resting. (Usual FS equivalents are combinations with more than two FS grade 3+.)
7.0	Unable to walk beyond about 5 metres even with aid, essentially restricted to wheelchair; wheels self in standard wheelchair and transfers alone; up and about in wheelchair some 12 hours a day. (Usual FS equivalents are combinations with more than one FS grade 4+; very rarely pyramidal grade 5 alone.)

(Continued)

Table 17.1 Kurtzke Expanded Disability Status Scale (EDSS) (*continued*)

Step	Description
7.5	Unable to take more than a few steps; restricted to wheelchair; may need aid in transfer; wheels self but cannot carry on in a standard wheelchair for a full day; may require a motorized wheelchair. (Usual FS equivalents are combinations with more than one FS grade 4+.)
8.0	Essentially restricted to bed or chair or perambulated in wheelchair but may be out of bed itself for much of the day; retains many self-care functions; generally has effective use of arms. (Usual FS equivalents are combinations, generally grade 4+ in several systems.)
8.5	Essentially restricted to bed much of the day; has some effective use of arm(s); retains some self-care functions. (Usual FS equivalents are combinations, generally 4+ in several systems.)
9.0	Helpless bed patient; can communicate and eat. (Usual FS equivalents are combinations, mostly grade 4+.)
9.5	Totally helpless bed patient; unable to communicate effectively or eat/swallow. (Usual FS equivalents are combinations, almost all grade 4+.)
10	Death due to MS

Disease-modifying treatment

There have recently been significant advances with regard to treatment possibilities for slowing down the progression of MS.

Corticosteroids

Adrenocorticosteroids have been used for many years for the treatment of relapse in MS. The best mode of steroid administration for relapse is intravenous methylprednisolone that can be quite safely given on an out-patient basis and in a single-bolus injection. There is no evidence that long-term steroid treatment has any effect on MS, and indeed it is probably detrimental in terms of undesirable steroid side-effects.

Azathioprine

There is some evidence that this is useful in reducing relapse rate, but is now used less often given the advent of interferon and other more effective therapies.

Cyclophosphamide

Cyclophosphamide is probably efficacious in the progressive phase of the disease, but there is little consensus on a suitable regimen. It is associated with significant side-effects.

Glatiramer acetate

This is a mixture of synthetic basic polypeptides and has recently become available for human use. It is given by daily subcutaneous injection. It is able to reduce the relapse rate and probably has a positive effect on long-term disability. It is usually well tolerated. In the UK there have been problems with prescription which is now restricted to recognized neurological treatment centres.

Interferons

- Interferon beta 1a
- Interferon beta 1b

Interferons are a group of naturally occurring proteins that modify the immune response. Interferon gamma appears to stimulate the immune response whereas interferons alpha and beta appear to be immunosuppressants. There have now been good quality and long-term studies that have shown efficacy of alpha and beta interferons in reducing the relapse rate and probably reducing long-term disability. This area has been controversial, and prescription is limited to specific neurological treatment centres. At the moment prescription is also limited to those who have relapsing/remitting disease under certain strict criteria. Each person put on interferon therapy in the UK has to be part of an on-going data collection trial that should confirm, or refute, the efficacy of these treatments over the next few years. The treatments are expensive (around £10 000 per annum per person). All the available compounds require subcutaneous injection. There is a range of troublesome side-effects, including local skin reactions, flu-like symptoms, and headache and a significant minority also seem to develop neutralizing antibodies which effectively stops clinical benefit. The interferons have also been shown to reduce lesion load on MRI scanning, which in theory should mean that there is less accumulating disability over time, but this point is not yet proven.

Natalizumab

- Approved by NICE in 2007 for patients with rapidly evolving severe relapsing-remitting forms of MS.
- Increases the numbers of circulating leukocytes due to inhibition of transmigration out of the vascular space. It is given IV every 4 weeks.
- Approved by the US FDA in November 2004 but withdrawn in February 2005 following reporting of 2 participants in clinical trials had developed progressive multifocal leukoencephalopathy (PML). In 2006 prescribing was resumed following a review of safety and effectiveness.
- Natalizumab has been shown to slow disability progression and in combinations with Interferon beta 1a reduced relapse rates by 50% compared to Interferon beta 1a alone.
- Because of the risk of PML, Tysabri is recommended for people who are not responding to their first line treatment.

Side effects

- PML.
- Infusion site reactions, fatigue, headaches, joint pain.
- Severe allergic reactions.
- Increased susceptibility to infections.

Other disease-modifying treatments

There have been many treatments that have come and gone in MS. Whilst some may have shown initial promise, such promise was not sustained after further studies. Other compounds have shown to have a beneficial effect but are associated with significant side effects. There are a few therapies worth a brief mention:

- *Hyperbaric oxygen*—this was in vogue in the 1970s but studies failed to support initial enthusiasm, although there may have been some improvement in bladder function and a suggestion of retardation of disease progression.
- *Diet*—the advantage of dietary manipulation is that the individual with MS feels that they are doing something for their own disease. Studies in the 1980s did demonstrate that a diet low in saturated fats and supplemented by N3 polyunsaturated fatty acids showed a non-significant trend towards shorter duration, reduced frequency, and severity of relapses. N3 fatty acids are found in fish oils.

Symptom management

Management of symptoms

There can be few disorders that require so much active interdisciplinary cooperation. The challenge for the rehabilitation team is to manage the complex interaction that lies behind disability, often involving several different neuronal systems. The complexity of the situation is illustrated by Table 17.2 which lists the symptoms in 656 people with MS.

Mobility

Difficulty walking is the most common symptom in MS. It is often due to a combination of different factors including:
- Pyramidal weakness.
- Spasticity.
- Fatigue.
- Disuse.
- Pain.
- Ataxia.
- Proprioceptive problems.

In the early stage a structured exercise programme, planned and supervised by a physiotherapist, can be of benefit. It has been recommended that the elements of such a programme should include:
- Specific strengthening exercises for identified muscle weakness.
- Exercises and advice on postural correction and control.
- Passive stretching to reduce spasticity, improve the range of movement, and prevent contractures.
- Exercises utilizing activities of daily living to improve dexterity and coordination.
- Gait training using mobility aids as necessary.
- Hydrotherapy to increase activity and range of movement dependent on the individual's reaction to heat as the hydrotherapy pool is kept at a temperature of 36° and this can induce fatigue.

It is likely that such an exercise programme will need to be continued for life but the availability of expert physiotherapy is sadly lacking for such long-term monitoring. However, if and when spasticity supervenes then the input of a physiotherapist is vital. The management of spasticity is covered elsewhere (🕮 see Chapter 6) but the following is a useful list of approaches to treatment:
- Reduction of external stimuli—e.g. catheter repositioning, foot care, bowel management, treatment of skin and urinary infections, etc.
- Physiotherapy, appropriate use of mobility aids and proper attention to seating and posture, both in wheelchair and leisure seating.
- Dynamic casting and correct use of orthoses, e.g. aircast splints, ankle foot orthoses.
- Pharmacological management, including peripheral nerve blocks and motor point blocks, botulinum toxin injections, and for more severe cases intrathecal baclofen or orthopaedic and neurosurgical procedures. If untreated, spasticity can easily lead to muscle contracture which in turn leads to worsening of posture, abnormal motor patterns, further pain, and an increased risk of pressure sores.

Table 17.2 Symptoms in 656 people with multiple sclerosis

Symptom present	No ADL difficulty (%)	With ADL difficulty (%)	Total (%)
Fatigue	21	56	77
Balance problems	24	50	74
Weakness or paralysis	18	45	63
Numbness, tingling, or other sensory disturbance	39	24	63
Bladder problems	25	34	59
Increased muscle tension (spasticity)	23	26	49
Bowel problems	19	20	39
Difficulty remembering	21	16	37
Depression	18	18	36
Pain	15	21	36
Laugh or cry easily (emotional lability)	24	8	32
Double or blurred vision, partial or complete blindness	14	16	30
Shaking (tremor)	14	13	27
Speech and/or communication difficulties	12	11	23
Difficulty solving problems	12	9	21

ADL, activities of daily living

From Kraft GH, Freal JE, and Coryll JK (1986). Disability, disease duration and rehabilitation service needs in multiple sclerosis: patient perspectives. *Archives of Physical Medicine and Rehabilitation*, **67**, 164–78

Upper limb function

Problems with arm functions are often a combination of pyramidal weakness combined with spasticity, ataxia, and sensory disturbance. In the case of arm difficulties an occupational therapist will need to be involved. The prescription of appropriate aids and equipment to daily living can be immensely helpful both to adapt the environment and for more immediate use by the individual. There is now a remarkable range of simple aids and equipment and adaptations that can make hand and arm tasks much simpler. There is some limited evidence that functionally orientated exercises utilizing simple daily living tasks can improve dexterity and coordination. Spasticity treatment in the arm is much more difficult than the leg, as the arm is less accessible to peripheral nerve blocks and much less amenable to surgical intervention.

Cerebellar dysfunction

Regrettably cerebellar involvement is common and also difficult to treat. There is little convincing evidence of a reliable improvement using any treatment. Specific drugs can sometimes be used with limited success, including:
- Isoniazid.
- Choline.
- Benzodiazepines.
- Sodium valproate.

Functional improvement will usually rest on the provision of adaptive equipment, such as:
- Large-handled implements.
- Plate guards.
- Velcro fastenings for buttons and shoelaces.
- Electric toothbrushes.
- Electric page turners, etc.

Occasionally severe intention tremor can be treated by cryothalamotomy or more recently by deep brain stimulation. Sometimes botulinum toxin can reduce very severe intention tremor but at the risk of generalized weakness.

Fatigue

Another of the most common symptoms in MS. It can have an over-whelming effect on daily activities and may be the main reason for reduced participation in terms of employment and leisure interests. The fatigue in MS can be secondary to depression or to the high energy cost of walking or other daily tasks. However, it seems that there is also a direct central mechanism for MS-related fatigue as there is only a poor correlation between fatiguability and physical disability.

Management of fatigue can be assisted by completion of a fatigue diary to identify if there are any patterns to fatigue and then making subsequent adjustments to lifestyle:
- Frequent rest periods throughout the day.
- Attention to sleep problems that may reduce daytime fatigue, such as the cautious and judicious use of short-acting benzodiazepines. The principle of 'little and often' is often the best way of managing fatigue.
- The use of anti-fatigue agents, such as amantadine, can also be helpful.

Swallowing disorders

Fortunately swallowing disorders are not that common except in very late stage MS. Swallowing disorders are discussed in Chapter 9 (⧉ see Management of swallowing disorders, p.136). In summary it is now recognized that swallowing is a highly complex motor sequence that requires expert evaluation by a speech and language therapist, dietician, and radiographer. Videofluroscopy is really the only way to make a proper assessment of dysphagia. However, there are a number of treatment possibilities for the different types of dysphagia. In later stage MS there is often an ethical problem with regard to swallowing disorders. How active should management be? In the author's view if, despite dietary manipulation, there are still difficulties with oral feeding and risk of malnutrition then a percutaneous endoscopic gastrostomy (PEG) tube should be considered sooner rather than later. This is a benign procedure and will usually improve quality of life.

Communication problems

Dysphasia is quite unusual in MS. The main problems of communication arise from dysarthria. Early referral to a speech and language therapist is important as there is evidence that early referral can improve functional communication abilities. Fortunately <1% of people with MS require augmentative communication aids but it is important to recognize the significant improvement in quality of life that can follow the prescription of such aids in this minority, i.e. LiteWriter.

Continence

Urinary problems are very common in MS. Urinary difficulties probably account for more handicap than any other problem. The commonest symptoms are:
- Urgency.
- Urge incontinence.
- Frequency.

These symptoms tend to be associated with bladder over-activity (detrusor hyper-reflexia). However, symptoms are not a reliable means of determining the underlying pathophysiology and urodynamics should be undertaken. About half the people with MS who have detrusor hyper-reflexia are also shown to have detrusor sphincter dyssynergia (☐ see Bladder detrusor-sphincter dyssynergia, p.112).

Less common symptoms are those often associated with bladder hypo-activity:
- Hesitancy.
- Overflow incontinence.
- Use of abdominal pressure when voiding.
- Episodes of retention.

These symptoms occur in about a quarter of those with MS with urinary symptoms.

Involvement of the upper urinary tract should now be unusual if there has been proper monitoring and urological follow-up. Whilst urodynamic assessment is important it is probably reasonable to offer anti-cholinergic medication on an empirical basis in the first instance if someone presents with frequency, urgency, and occasional urge incontinence. First choice is probably oxybutynin (dose 2.5–3mg twice a day increasing to a maximum of 5mg three times a day). Other possibilities are tolterodine (dose 2mg twice daily, propantheline bromide and imipramine. If this medication is not sufficient then urodynamic assessment is required.

Intermittent catheterization has markedly improved management for many people. Residual post-micturition volume should be ascertained, preferably by ultrasound, although post-micturition catheterization is a reasonable alternative. If the residual volume is >100mL this is probably an indication for catheterization. Intermittent catheterization either by the patient or by a third party is the first choice. However, weakness, incoordination, adductor spasticity, or unavailability of a suitable carer can still necessitate an indwelling catheter. Suprapubic catheterization has been shown to be much safer, with less risk of infection, than urethral catheterization.

Most people are able to manage their urinary symptoms by a combination of anti-cholinergic medication and intermittent catheterization—only around 10% need more specialist urological referral and treatment. Appropriate use should be made of the specialist nurse continence advisors that are now widely available throughout the UK. These individuals can provide practical advice on aids and appliances as well as psychological support and counselling.

Bowel problems

Constipation can occur in many people with MS. Fortunately faecal incontinence is less common, although faecal overflow can occur in the context of constipation. The situation is usually resolved by:
- Attention to both timing and amount of time spent in defaecation.
- Maximal use of gastric colic reflex.
- Appropriate use of mechanical factors, such as hip flexion during defaecation.
- Abdominal pressure or digital stimulation can be helpful.
- A diet high in fibre supplemented, if needed, by bulking agents with adequate water intake.
- If the above measures fail then other medication can be used, such as sodium docusate, laxatives, and enemas.

Sexual function

In one study three-quarters of the men and over half of the women had sexual problems in the context of MS. In women this mainly was secondary to:
- Fatigue.
- Decreased sensation.
- Decreased libido.
- Problems with orgasm.

In men fatigue and decreased libido were also problems but they also had difficulty in achieving and maintaining erection.

The management of sexual difficulties is a specialist field and if possible referral to an appropriate sexual advisory service for people with disabilities should be made. Sexual counselling and treatment can consist of the following:
- Straightforward practical advice, such as the best time for intercourse with regard to fatigue.
- Optimization of medication.
- Correct advice on bladder management.
- Advice on positioning.

Adductor spasticity can be a particular problem which may be helped by physiotherapy or nerve blocks. Erectile dysfunction in the male is now usually treated by sildenafil. If sildenafil cannot be tolerated then male erectile dysfunction can be helped by self-injection of papaverine. Other techniques include vacuum condom and venostricture devices and sometimes the use of penile prostheses, but the latter techniques have now been largely superseded by the use of sildenafil.

The main point to emphasize is for sexuality to be viewed in its broadest context—only part of which is penetrative sexual intercourse.

There is no evidence that fertility is impaired in MS.

Pain and paroxysmal symptoms

Pain can be a real difficulty in MS. Around half of people have an acute or chronic pain problem. Some people have acute paroxysmal pain including:

- Trigeminal neuralgia.
- L'Hermitte's syndrome (pain on neck flexion).
- Paroxysmal burning pain.
- Painful tonic seizures.

These paroxysmal painful syndromes respond well to anti-convulsant medication such as carbamazepine or gabapentin.

Longer-term pain can be due to a variety of causes, including:

- Musculoskeletal pain secondary to posture disturbance, such as wheelchair dependency giving rise to low back pain or shoulder pain secondary to self-propelling of the wheelchair.
- Chronic neuralgic pain, probably secondary to the disease process itself—this can respond to carbamazepine and/or gabapentin.
- Pain from spasticity, which can respond to anti-spastic measures, particularly botulinum toxin; this can also act as an analgesic as well as an anti-spastic agent.

Visual disturbance

Optic neuritis is one of the main presenting symptoms of MS and will often respond well to corticosteroid therapy. However, there are a range of other problems including:

- Residual scotomas.
- Diplopia.
- Oscillopsia.

Many such symptoms are difficult to treat. Symptomatic nystagmus can be helped by converging prisms or botulinum toxin therapy. Referral to low-vision clinics can sometimes be necessary and helpful.

General medical problems

There are a whole variety of other general medical difficulties that can arise in MS. These would include:

- Pressure sores.
- Peripheral oedema.
- Deep venous thrombosis—but fortunately people with MS seem to have a low risk.
- Heterotopic ossification—but also rare in MS.
- Hearing problems—very rare in MS.

Cognitive dysfunction

Intellectual impairment was recognized by the earliest describers of MS, such as Charcot and l'Hermitte. In modern practice cognitive problems have tended to be under-emphasized. However, there is no doubt that cognitive impairment can be detected even in the early stages of MS. The commonest problems are:

- Memory difficulties.
- Problems with information processing speed—the individual may appear 'slow on the uptake'.
- Retrograde learning.

Some recommend brief screening tests, such as the Mini Mental State Examination or the Screening Examination for Cognitive Impairment (SEFCI), which can be useful as an aid to deciding who to refer to for a more complete neuropsychological assessment. Preferably a clinical neuropsychologist should be an integral part of any MS rehabilitation team.

Emotional problems

- Depression occurs in up to 50% of the MS population at some point. There is no evidence that depression in the context of MS responds any differently from other depressive illness and should be treated appropriately (📖 see p.202).
- Clinical anxiety is a further problem which is often made worse by lack of proper information or time for simple counselling and support. The MS literature refers to euphoria being quite common, although this does seem to be a most unusual symptom.
- A small number of people develop emotionalism (see Emotionalism, p.210) which responds well to a small dose of a tricyclic anti-depressant.

Participation issues

Problems in MS can often be unnecessarily compounded by a lack of knowledge regarding local services and facilities. Health professionals in the rehabilitation team should be acquainted with:

- Local accessible leisure pursuits.
- Day centre provision.
- Respite care provision.
- How to access local housing and housing adaptation systems.
- Welfare rights services.
- Employment rehabilitation services.
- Carer support groups.
- Information and advice services.
- Contact address of local and national MS societies and other self-help groups.

It is particularly important to emphasize employment rehabilitation. This can be a major concern amongst the MS population as the disease mainly affects those of working age. About 80% of the economic loss to the national economy from people with MS is accounted for by lost earnings. The unemployment rate in most studies is very high and usually exceeds 50%.

Service delivery

There is now good evidence that access to a skilled multidisciplinary rehabilitation team can make a real impact on the lives of people with MS. Studies have shown that a brief period (around 2 weeks) of inpatient admission to a rehabilitation unit can improve activity and participation even in the context of worsening impairment. However, it is probable that such benefits may be lost over time if there is no long-term support. Individuals with MS should preferably have access to the rehabilitation team on a regular basis—even if this just involves simple telephone advice or self-referral at times of problems. A formal regular review is probably needed in order to prevent unnecessary or unrecognized complications from arising. Evidence in Newcastle upon Tyne showed that the costs of introducing a community-based MS team were matched by the reduction in costs from unnecessary hospital admissions, outpatient referrals, and reduction in GP contact time.

The needs of the MS family focus on the following:
- *Time*—to discuss diagnosis and treatment as well as more personal cognitive and emotional difficulties. A counsellor attached to the MS team is a valuable asset.
- *Information*—at the time of diagnosis and in the longer term to keep up to date with research and potential treatments.
- *Practical help*—in terms of the provision of aids and equipment as well as access to personal help within the home.
- *Carer's need*—an equal need for access to information and counselling support as well as the need for access to respite facilities.

The recent development of a network of MS nurse specialists has been a welcome addition to community support. The nurses are well trained and can deal with many daily problems in MS and also act as a source of referral to more specialist support. Every individual with MS should have access to an MS nurse specialist and preferably access to a specialist rehabilitation team.

Further reading

1. www.msif.org/en/—provides independent information from MS professionals worldwide.
2. www.mssociety.org.uk/for_professionals/resources—the website of the MS society which provides an excellent resource for those with MS and their families and also healthcare professionals.
3. http://www.nice.org.uk/guidance/CG8—NICE guidelines for MS, 2003. NICE guidelines provided on this website.
4. www.mstrust.org.uk—provides information for people with MS, their families and healthcare professionals.

Stroke

Definition

A stroke is an injury to the brain, following an interruption to the normal cerebral circulation resulting in the onset of neurological loss over a short period of time. It is known as a cerebrovascular accident and may follow either an intracerebral haemorrhage, a cerebral infarction or a subarachnoid haemorrhage. There is a need to distinguish these three because there are different factors in primary and secondary prevention and some differing rehabilitative needs. Subarachnoid haemorrhage (in contrast to cerebral infarction and haemorrhage) often presents with more global deficits producing significant cognitive as well as physical problems. Transient cerebral ischaemic attack (or mini-stroke) is defined by symptoms lasting for not more than 24 hours. There is agreement that early intervention does bring benefits, both in terms of mortality and morbidity.

Epidemiology

- *Incidence*—common: 200/100000 population.
- *Prevalence*—550/100000 population; 400 with significant disability per 250,000 population.
- *Mortality*—30% in first month, 40% in first year. Myocardial infarction, bronchopneumonia and further stroke commonest causes.
- *Disability*—50% weakness, 15–20% dysphasia, 10% cognitive deficit (memory, perception, intellect, and other higher cerebral functioning).

Classification and diagnosis

- Transient ischaemic attack.
- Subarachnoid haemorrhage.
- Intracerebral haemorrhage.
- Infarction:
  - Total anterior circulation infarct.
  - Partial anterior circulation infarct.
  - Lacunar infarct (Box 18.1).
  - Posterior circulation infarct.

The impairments resulting from stroke depend on the location of the lesion.

Box 18.1 Lacunar infarcts

These are often multiple and result from occlusion of small arteries of 50–150mm in diameter. They are associated with hypertension and arteriosclerosis and give rise to multiple, deep, small cavities, known as lacunae. They produce four specific syndromes which are as follows:
- Hemiparesis with ataxia affecting the leg more than the arm—from an infarct in the internal capsule.
- Pure motor hemiplegia—from an infarct in the pons or internal capsule.
- Dysarthria–clumsy hand syndrome (pons)—dysarthria, slight dysphagia, central facial weakness, deviation of tongue to affected side and clumsiness and ataxia in ipsilateral hand to side of lesion.
- Pure sensory stroke with unilateral sensory loss for all modalities of sensation—posterolateral thalamic nucleus infarct.

More rare syndromes, e.g. lateral medullary syndromes, can be found in more detail in a neurology text.

Anatomy and localizing features of brain disease (Table 18.1)

Visual loss in stroke is shown in Fig. 18.1.

Table 18.1 Impairment/deficit according to the site of the brain lesion

Site	Impairments/deficits
Frontal lobe	Behavioural abnormalities
	Planning/anticipatory difficulties
	Inertia and decreased initiative
Parietal lobe	Spatial disorientation
	Apraxia
	Agnosia
	Sensory inattention
	Receptive dysphasia**
	Homonymous hemianopia*
Pre-central gyrus (in parietal lobe)	Localized weakness/monoplegia
	Expressive dysphasia*
Post central gyrus	Localized sensory loss
Temporal lobe	Memory
	Hallucination (auditory and visual)
	Decreased concentration/attention
	Receptive dysphasia
	Quadratic hemianopia
Occipital lobe	Hemianopia
Base of brain	Hemiplegia and hemi-anaesthesia
	Spasticity ++ cranial nerve deficits
Brain stem	Ataxia
	Cranial nerve problems, particularly dysarthria and diplopia
	Spasticity +++
	Diffuse (as found in SAH)
	Decreased information processing
	Decreased IQ
	Cognitive problems

*Dominant hemisphere; **non-dominant hemisphere. SAH subarachnoid haemorrhage.

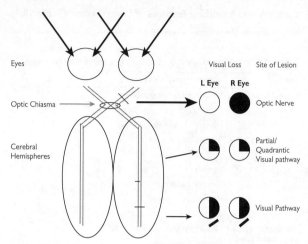

Fig. 18.1 Visual loss in stroke

Investigations

The completed stroke

Urgent CT scans are performed to determine the site and size of the lesion

CT scans are normal in about 15% of cases. They actually rarely change the management of the patient, but are essential in four specific situations.

- To exclude cerebral haemorrhage when anti-coagulant or anti-platelet treatment is being considered.
- When there is a suspicion that a patient has an intracranial mass due to tumour, subdural haematoma, or abscess.
- When intracranial hypertension is suspected, particularly if the patient's level of consciousness is dropping and surgical intervention is being considered.
- When the patient's course is atypical and the diagnosis is in doubt.

All other investigations are directed to:

- Exclude other causes of the acute stroke syndrome.
- Reveal some underlying cause for the stroke, or
- Detect some potential complication of a stroke.

Differential

- Tumours/subdural haematoma—seek surgical advice.
- Post epileptic paresis—non-specific change in consciousness.
- Biochemical abnormalities—require investigation; rarely cause stroke.
- Myocardial disease—cardiac assessment important. Anti-coagulants for atrial fibrillation in absence of cerebral haemorrhage.

Transient ischaemic attacks (TIAs)

TIAs require full investigation in order to prevent completed strokes

Management centres on reducing the risk factors (hypertension, smoking, diabetes and other rarer abnormalities, e.g. anaemia, polycythaemia).

Look for:

- Arrhythmias.
- Significant carotid artery occlusion—treatable by endarterectomy.
- Reducing risk factors by health education:
  - Cessation of smoking.
  - Weight reduction in obese people.
  - Lipid reduction.
  - Diabetic control.
  - Increasing physical activity.

Rehabilitation of the completed stroke patient

There is no such thing as a 'simple stroke', since neither the disabilities nor the patient's circumstances are ever straightforward. Each patient needs individual consideration within a standard plan for assessment.

Medical assessment

A comprehensive history (which may have to be provided by a relative in patients with communication or cognitive problems) and examination to identify impairments, functioning, and potential for participation.

- Physical and nutritional status.
- Motor and sensory deficits, including visual field defects, dysaesthesia, and paraesthesiae.
- Incontinence.
- Tissue viability problems.
- Spasticity.
- Dysphagia (due to poor bulbar function).
- Communication difficulties.
- Cognitive deficits and mood.
- The patient's domestic situation and social history.
- The health of carers and their ability to carry out care functions.
- Pre-existing and comorbid disease, which may act as a barrier to successful rehabilitation.

Special points in assessment

History taking and examination (Box 18.2) are important, not only for identifying prognostic factors, but for providing medical input into the rehabilitation process.

> **Box 18.2 Suggested headings for history taking and examination**
>
> - Motor function
> - Sensation
> - Vision
> - Swallowing
> - Communication
> - Higher cerebral functions
> - Other problems

Formal measurement is important and this is addressed in Chapter 5.
- *Motor function*—assess dexterity and shoulder function, the ability to initiate movements, grip, pinch grip, ability to raise the hand to the mouth or occiput, walking speed (10-metre walking time), Ashworth score.
- *Swallowing*—time taken to drink 150mL of water. If there is any choking, the test should be aborted immediately and suction should always be at hand to deal with any problems. People with normal swallowing functions can usually manage this quantity of fluid within 10–12 seconds.

- *Vision*—formal visual field test by perimetry should be undertaken when visual loss is suspected.
- *Communication*—see p.144.

Predictors of prognostication (Table 18.2)

Table 18.2 Prognostic indicators

Early mortality at onset	Capillary abnormalities
	Gaze paresis
	Abnormal respiratory pattern
	Bilateral extensor plantar responses
	Persistence of hypertension and significant cardiac disease
Poor signs at 1 week	MRC grade 0 power in upper limb
	Unable to locate affected thumb with eyes closed
	Cannot maintain sitting balance
	Incontinence
	Loss of consciousness at onset
Prognosticators of poor functional outcome at 4 weeks post-stroke	Low scores in the Barthel scale of activities of daily living (ADL)
	Pre-existing and post-stroke incontinence
Adverse factors	Inability to walk
	Loss of arm function
	Loss of postural control
	Hemianopia
	Proprioceptive sensory loss
	Spatial neglect
	Impaired cognition
Rate limiting barriers in rehabilitation	Pre-existing physical disability (e.g. joint or cardiopulmonary disease)
	Multiple pathology (e.g. loss of limb)
	Sensory impairment
	Complications of disabling disease
	Incontinence
	Pressure sores
	Impairment of intellect, memory, perception, communication, mood
Signs for good outcome	Reverse of poor prognostic signs
	Early return of hand movement and shoulder protraction (return of prehensile function and ADL)
	Youth, and a motivation to achieve realistic targets

Social circumstances—socio-economic class, wealth, home ownership and a good supportive family—can affect the chance of a patient living at home, but they are not, somewhat strangely, indicators per se of a good prognosis in terms of independent living. Good cognition and communication and the ability to move the thumb and the foot are better.

Higher cerebral functions (Table 18.3)

Table 18.3 Assessment of higher cerebral functions

Cognitive disorder	Appropriate bedside test
Orientation	Hodkinson's test
Memory	Mini-Mental State Examination
Perception	Rivermead behavioural inattention test (star cancellation, line crossing)
Apraxias:	
Ideomotor	Miming simple action, e.g. whistling, combing hair, smiling, waving
Ideational	More complex tasks such as miming, lighting candle or cigarette, opening door
Constructional	Drawings, building blocks etc. (pick 5 standard tasks for each problem and simple scores can be derived)
Numeracy and intellect	Serial sevens—subtraction from 100
	Require detailed thorough examination by a clinical psychologist, e.g. IQ, using WAIS-R scale.

Special problems
- Incontinence, constipation and pressure sores.
- Pressure sores, check the skin regularly.
- Side-effects of medical treatments.
- Spasticity is a major issue in stroke.
- Depression.

Further reading
1. Warlow CP, Dennis MS, Van Gijn K, et al. (2001). *Stroke: A Practical Guide to Management*. Blackwell Science, Oxford.
2. Wade D (1992). *Measurement in Neurological Disability*. Oxford University Press, Oxford.

Chapter 19

Traumatic brain injury

Background and epidemiology

Head injury is one of the most challenging disorders faced by the rehabilitation team. An individual with traumatic brain injury will often have a complex range of physical, behavioural, emotional, cognitive, and social problems. However, there is now good evidence that a multidisciplinary rehabilitation team can make a real difference to outcome and that such a team is clearly preferable to management on a general medical or surgical ward. Regrettably few people in the UK or elsewhere in the world yet have access to such a team. Most people receive good-quality immediate neurosurgical care but most are then discharged back to the local district general hospital or straight back home without any rehabilitation support or follow-up. There are now a few regional specialist neurological rehabilitation centres that cater for such individuals but they are still insufficient to cater for the needs of all those with severe brain injury, let alone those with moderate or milder problems. More importantly there are very few good quality community head injury teams that work with the person after the acute phase when they have returned home.

The annual attendance rate at casualty departments with a traumatic brain injury is around 1500–2000 per 100 000 population per annum. Obviously the majority of these people have a minor head injury. Around 10% have a moderate head injury and about 5% a severe head injury. Formal definition of these categories is given in Table 19.1.

A traumatic brain injury can be seen as a chain of events. The first injury occurs in the seconds after the event; the second injury in the minutes and hours following, depending on when medical intervention takes place. The third injury and time following the above two can cause further injuries.

- There are three sorts of first injury:
  - Closed injury—often happens with rapid acceleration/deceleration.
  - Open or penetrating injury, e.g. bullet wound.
  - Crush injury, e.g. road traffic accident.
- Second injury—due to hypoxia.
- Third injury—could be as a result of bleeding, bruising, or swelling in the brain.

The majority of brain injuries are secondary to road traffic accidents, with a smaller proportion due to domestic or industrial accidents, sporting injuries, or violence. Prevalence is thought to be around 100–150 individuals with persistent disability as a result of traumatic brain injury per 100 000 population.

Table 19.1 Classification of head injury

Classification	Definition
Mild head injury	GCS13 or 14 *or* coma <15 minutes
Moderate head injury	GCS 8–12 with coma between 15 minutes–6 hours *or* post-traumatic amnesia <24 hours
Severe head injury	GCS <7 *or* coma >6 hours *or* post-traumatic amnesia >24 hours

GCS Glasgow Coma Scale

Glasgow Coma Scale

The GCS is the most widely used scoring system, used in quantifying the level of consciousness of a patient following traumatic brain injury. It provides a score in the range of 3–15 with the lowest possible score being 3. It probably reflects the severity of brain injury and there is a correlation between the GCS score and eventual outcome; the lower the score the worse the eventual outcome. The GCS is given in Table 19.2.[1–3]

References

1. Teasdale, G and Jennett B (1974). Assessment of coma and impaired consciousness. A practical scale. *Lancet*, **2**, 81–3.
2. Teasdale G, Knill-Jones R, and Van der Sande J (1978). Observer variability in assessing impaired consciousness and coma. *Journal of Neurology, Neurosurgery and Psychiatry*, **41**, 603–10.
3. Teasdale G, Murray G, Parker L, *et al.* (1979). Adding up the Glasgow Coma Scale. *Acta Neurochirurgica*, **28** (Suppl.), 13–16.

Table 19.2 GCS[1–3]

Item	Response	Score	Details
Eye opening	None	1	Even to pain (supra-orbital pressure)
	To pain	2	Pain from sternum/limb/supra-orbital ridge pressure
	To speech	3	Non-specific response, not necessarily to command
	Spontaneous	4	Eyes open, not necessarily aware
Motor response	None	1	To any pain; limbs remain flaccid
	Extension	2	'Decerebrate'; shoulder adducted and internally rotated, forearm pronated
	Abnormal flexion	3	'Decorticate'; shoulder flexes/adducts
	Withdrawal	4	Arm withdraws from pain, shoulder abducts
	Localizes pain	5	Arm attempts to remove supra-orbital/chest pressure
	Obeys commands	6	Follows simple commands
Verbal response	None	1	As stated
	Incomprehensible	2	Moans/groans; no words
	Inappropriate	3	Intelligible, no sustained sentences
	Confused	4	Responds with conversation, but confused
	Oriented	5	Aware of time, place, person

Prognosis

There is no accurate way of determining prognosis in traumatic brain injury. Certain clear generalizations are possible:

- The lower the initial GCS score the worse the outcome.
- The longer the coma the worse the outcome.
- The longer the period of post-traumatic amnesia the worse the outcome. (The latter is defined as the period of time from injury until resumption of day-to-day memory.)
- There is a crude correlation between the amount of brain damage (as determined by MRI scanning) and long-term outlook.

However, there are many exceptions to these general rules and it is always unwise to give any definite prognosis within the first few weeks of injury.

Most physical recovery will occur in the first 12 months, but some physical improvement can certainly occur during the second year after injury. Neuropsychological recovery takes much longer and between 2 and 3 years is usually taken as a reasonable length of time for natural recovery to continue. After this period of time, once natural recovery has been completed, functional improvements can still occur by development of appropriate coping strategies and support mechanisms.

Life expectancy is usually normal after head injury except for people with severe disabilities. There are generally agreed to be five factors that reduce life expectancy in traumatic brain injury and indeed in the disabled population as a whole. These are:

- Immobility.
- Incontinence.
- Inability to swallow and consequent necessity of tube or percutaneous endoscopic gastrostomy (PEG) feeding.
- On-going and uncontrolled epilepsy.
- Severe cognitive and intellectual damage.

There are some early indications that after traumatic brain injury individuals may have a higher risk of dementia in later life. However, this is still controversial and such a link is by no means definite.

Minor head injury

The great majority of people with a minor, or even a moderate, head injury make an excellent recovery over a few days or after a week or so. However, there is a significant minority (probably around 10%) of people with minor head injury who continue to have long-term problems over many months or even in the long term. In the past such symptoms have been called 'post-concussional' but such a blanket label is probably best avoided. It is better to annotate each separate symptom in order to determine whether anything can be done about each individual problem. Some of the commoner 'post-concussional' symptoms are:

- Headaches.
- Dizziness.
- Insomnia.
- Fatigue.
- Poor concentration.
- Mild memory disturbance/forgetfulness.
- Slowed ability to learn and process new information.
- Anxiety.
- Depression.
- Irritability.
- Sleep disturbance.

These problems can be cumulative following repeated minor head injury, which may account for some of the longer-term problems encountered in, for example, boxing or horse racing.

It is now generally accepted that such problems are organic in nature rather than related to psychological factors such as coping style or symptom exaggeration in the context of litigation.

In an ideal world everyone with a minor head injury should be followed up at least once after around 3 months in order to identify those who are more likely to have persistent problems. Those individuals may need longer-term counselling and support or perhaps specific interventions, such as full neuropsychological assessment and a cognitive remediation programme.

It is likely that symptoms can be reduced by proper information being given at the time of the head injury at discharge from casualty. A series of booklets on head injury, and in particular mild head injury, produced by the Headway charity are useful in this regard.[1] Contact could be made with the local Headway group for further peer support.

It is regrettably common that people with minor head injury return to work too soon and find that they have difficulty coping with their job. Proper information and advice, not only to the head-injured person but also the employer and the person's family, is vital.

Regrettably there are very few mild head injury clinics in the UK or indeed worldwide.

References
1. ⌀ www.headway.org.uk—website of the charity headway in the UK.

Organization of services

There are a number of stages to proper care of individuals after traumatic brain injury.

Stage 1: immediate trauma care

Fast emergency care and appropriate road-side treatment are important followed by rapid transfer to the nearest trauma centre for stabilization. Such centres should be in close association with the neurosurgical unit with access to MRI scanning and cerebral pressure monitoring. Occasionally neurosurgical intervention will be necessary for evacuation of blood clots, elevation of depressed skull fracture, etc. The rehabilitation team should be associated with the acute neurosurgical team. There are a number of complications that can arise in the first few hours and days after injury which if dealt with properly can prevent major rehabilitation difficulties later. An example would be active intervention for spasticity in order to prevent contractures, and assessment of swallowing with appropriate initiation of gastrostomy feeding.

Stage 2: post-acute rehabilitation

As soon as the individual is surgically and medically stable they should be transferred to the nearest specialist head injury rehabilitation centre. Regrettably there are few such centres in the UK and many people bypass this stage. There is now clear evidence that post-acute brain injury rehabilitation produces better functional outcome. The sooner the transfer is made to the rehabilitation unit the better the outcome.

Stage 3: 'step-down' rehabilitation

Most people with severe brain injury will make rapid progress over the first few months after the accident. However, after around 6 months progress will begin to plateau. At this time they still have further rehabilitation potential and sometimes transfer to a 'step-down' rehabilitation unit is appropriate. This is a step towards discharge home and such a unit may concentrate on smooth staged discharge back into the home environment. Such a unit is usually most appropriate when there are delays to being transferred home, such as the need for home adaptations. Alternatively individuals with severe cognitive and intellectual damage or behavioural disturbance may need a much more prolonged period of rehabilitation in a less acute environment. Many individuals will bypass this stage and move straight back home.

Stage 4: community-based rehabilitation

Obviously it is the eventual aim that everyone returns home after traumatic brain injury. Sometimes this is not possible, but nevertheless the great majority of people should be able to get back to their home and family. There is good evidence that the most significant problems for the family and carers occur after discharge home and at this stage long-term support is essential. This should consist of on-going home-based rehabilitation by a multidisciplinary team. Often a care manager is required to coordinate the complex range of services that are required. Physiotherapists, occupational therapists, speech and language therapists, clinical psychologists, medical staff, and social service staff can still need to be involved. Long-term emotional support both to the disabled person and the family is often required. Regrettably there are few coordinated community based rehabilitation teams in the UK or elsewhere.

Thus, there are regrettably very few people who go through a proper staged rehabilitation process after traumatic brain injury. This is a pity as there is now good evidence of the efficacy of a staged multidisciplinary rehabilitation programme.

Each stage should not be seen as a self-contained entity as liaison will still be needed between the staff in the acute rehabilitation unit and, for example, the community team. Staff sharing is often appropriate. Sometimes individuals will need referral back to a specialist centre for management of particular problems, such as PEG feeding or spasticity management. Occasionally referral needs to be made to a specialist subunit, such as a unit catering for people with severe behavioural disturbance.

Physical disability

Severe physical disability following brain injury is quite uncommon. The brain appears to have a remarkable capacity for functional recovery even after quite severe injury. However, a whole range of physical problems are obviously possible after brain trauma. The commonest problems are:

- Walking problems—usually secondary to either spasticity, weakness, or ataxia but often there is a multifactorial causation (🕮 see Chapter 6).
- Problems with daily living tasks secondary to similar difficulties in the arms.
- Communication problems secondary to dysarthria or dysphasia (🕮 see Chapter 10).
- Swallowing problems often secondary to brainstem damage. PEG feeding is commonly required in severe brain injury at least for the first few months (🕮 see Management of swallowing problems, p.136).
- Continence problems—usually secondary to detrusor hyper-reflexia or sometimes to detrusor sphincter dyssynergia (🕮 see Management of urinary problems, p.114; Detrusor sphincter dyssynergia, p.112).
- Visual disturbance—blindness, diplopia, or visual neglect.
- Sensory disturbance often compounded by sensory neglect, although this is more common after focal cerebral lesions, such as stroke.
- Loss of the sense of smell is very common even in minor head injuries.
- Post-traumatic epilepsy (see the next section).

Obviously many of these problems are amenable to rehabilitation intervention. Treatment for these various symptoms are described in other chapters of this book.

Post-traumatic epilepsy

Epilepsy after traumatic brain injury is more common if:

- There is a depressed skull fracture.
- There has been intracranial haemorrhage.
- There is clear focal brain damage as opposed to diffuse axonal injury.
- Later epilepsy is common if there has been an epileptic seizure within the first week after injury.

There are tables that indicate the risk of epilepsy according to the presence or absence of these risk factors. If no risk factors are present then the risk of post-traumatic epilepsy is relatively small at only about 2–3%. Many authorities would not initiate prophylactic anti-convulsant medication unless there is a very high risk of epilepsy. Carbamazepine is probably the anti-convulsant of first choice in epilepsy secondary to traumatic brain injury.

Minimally conscious and vegetative states

Around 1% of people after head injury remain in a prolonged coma (defined as a coma of >2 weeks' duration). About half of those who remain in a coma at 1 month have regained consciousness by 3 months although overall functional outlook for this group remains poor. Less than 10% of those recovering from coma that has lasted up to 3 months return to any form of employment. The longer individuals remain comatose the poorer the outcome. Life expectancy is clearly reduced in those with prolonged coma, although there are cases of individuals surviving many years in such a state. Survival is usually dependent on continuing high-quality nursing care, particularly avoidance of pressure sores and active treatment of infections as well as continuing nutrition, usually by PEG feeding.

The SMART[1,2]—sensory modality and assessment rehabilitation technique—is now being used in specialist regional services to assess awareness in adults who have sustained profound brain damage and been diagnosed as in vegetative state (VS) or minimally conscious (MCS).

- It can identify the full range of the patient's functional and communication capabilities.
- This to date is the only tool currently available which has been specifically designed to provide a series of sensory assessments over time to identify awareness.
- It studies the patient's response to a multi-sensory programme including vision, hearing, taste, touch, and smell. Modalities of wakefulness/arousal, motor skills, and functional communication are also thoroughly assessed.
- Following assessment a SMART treatment programme can then be instigated followed by a further re-assessment.
- The programme is designed by the outcome of the assessment. It utilizes selected modalities of the assessment and incorporates familiar and unfamiliar stimuli to produce a programme to meet the patient's specific requirements.

Difficult ethical issues arise when the treating rehabilitation team and the family are agreed that active treatment should be withdrawn. In the UK such decisions are now taken by the Court. The family and the treating physician will need to be in agreement. An independent medical expert is appointed both for the patient and also for the hospital and family. Solicitors are also appointed on both sides in order to make sure there is no major financial advantage that would accrue to a third party following the patient's death. The expert reports are presented to a judge who will make a final decision. Euthanasia remains illegal in most countries but withdrawal of active treatment, such as withdrawal of feeding, is allowable after appropriate Court approval.

Great care must be taken in making a diagnosis of persistent or permanent vegetative state. One study indicated a misdiagnosis rate of 40%. Some individuals seem to retain some awareness which is difficult to access and only becomes apparent after detailed and prolonged observation. Deafness and/or visual problems also seem quite common in those with prolonged coma which makes proper assessment even more difficult. The quality of life of people in prolonged coma is probably maximized by transfer to a specialist MCS or VS unit. Regrettably there are very few such units in the UK or worldwide.

References

1. ☝ www.rhn.org.uk/institute—the Institute of Neuropalliative Rehabilitiation website.
2. Gill-Thwaites H and Munday R (1999). The sensory modality assessment rehabilitation technique (SMART): A comprehensive and integrated assessment and treatment protocol of the vegetative state and minimally responsive patient. *Neuropsychological Rehabilitation*, **9**, 305–20.

Cognitive problems

There are a large variety of important cognitive and intellectual problems that follow traumatic brain injury. The assessment and treatment of these conditions is covered in more detail in Chapter 15 (📖 Cognitive and intellectual function, p.213). The commonest problems are:

- Problems with recent memory.
- Difficulties with concentration and attention.
- Slowed learning speed and reduced information-processing speed.
- Poor initiation.
- Difficulties with planning, often needing someone else to prompt and guide the person even for simple daily living tasks.
- Problem solving.
- Perceptual problems—often visual or sensory neglect.
- Problems with topographical orientation and naming problems.
- Communication problems, particularly dysphasia and dysarthria.

Rehabilitation depends on accurate assessment, which should be carried out by a clinical neuropsychologist. Such assessment needs to not only document the areas of impairment but also the areas of relatively intact function which can be used to form an appropriate coping strategy.

There is now emerging evidence that various cognitive strategies can produce improvements in quality of life and real functional improvements in the clinic setting can generalize back at home. Some brain injury rehabilitation units now have specific cognitive clinics where such people can be assessed and coping strategies planned and enacted.

The use of simple memory aids, diaries, pagers, and the use of mnemonics can, for example, produce significant benefit for those with memory problems (📖 see Cognitive rehabilitation, p.226).

Behavioural and emotional problems

Behavioural problems

Behavioural problems are very common in the early recovery phase following brain injury. Patients may present in post-traumatic amnesia (PTA). This is defined as 'the inability to remember continuous events, after a blow to the head, which causes an alteration of consciousness even when the patient is apparently awake'. Symptoms are loss of memory for the present time; confusion and agitation; violence and aggression; and disinhibition.

At this stage sedative and psychotropic medication should be avoided if at all possible. Such drugs simply add to the confusion and general clouding of consciousness. This in turn can cause more behavioural disturbance leading to a vicious circle. At this stage individuals are often best nursed in separate rooms with quiet surroundings and lack of sensory stimulation. Some brain injury units now have a PTA room in order to nurse such people.

A small number of people develop longer-term behavioural difficulties after brain injury which can amount to significant verbal and physical aggression. Behavioural management techniques are known to be effective in ameliorating such problems. Such techniques are often best put into place in specialist units so that all staff and relatives can cooperate in a strict behavioural regimen. The nature of behavioural management programmes has been described in Chapter 13 (📖 see p. 192).

Emotional problems

After brain injury it is common to hear relatives complain that 'he is not the person I married' or 'it is like living with a different person'. However, the term 'personality change' should be avoided. It is better to document the details of any perceived change in order that appropriate strategies can be designed to alleviate the problem. There are many such changes and the commonest are:

• Childish or fatuous behaviour.
• Egocentricity.
• Irritability.
• Aggression.
• Lack of initiation and reduced drive.
• Lethargy.
• Lack of social skills.
• Increased or decreased sexual interest.

These problems cause family and work disruption after the person has returned home. Many families can cope with residual physical problems but find such subtle personality changes very difficult to manage.

Such changes are difficult to ameliorate and there is often little that can be done except offer counselling or psychotherapy to support the family. Sometimes a behavioural programme can improve the situation, particularly with regard to irritability or aggression. It is often surprisingly difficult to help the problems of reduced drive and lack of initiative.

Clinical depression or clinical anxiety are also quite common at some point during the recovery phase and are said to occur in around 50% of both head-injured people and carers. These problems often occur soon after return home and once again this emphasizes the need for support at this time. Occasionally profound psychiatric problems can emerge such as psychosis, mania, or obsessive compulsive disorder either in a previously predisposed individual or perhaps as a result of direct organic brain damage. The involvement of a neuropsychiatrist is important in such cases. Depression and anxiety also need active and sometimes aggressive treatment.

Later-stage rehabilitation

The previous sections in this chapter have emphasized the importance of long-term community-based support. Discharge from the rehabilitation centre will often occur after a few months and there can be many months of further natural recovery requiring an active rehabilitation programme. Even if natural recovery has ceased then there is still a need for support to avoid the emergence of unnecessary physical, cognitive, intellectual, behavioural, and emotional complications.

Independent living skills and social skills

There is emerging evidence of the efficacy of specific training programmes for independent living skills, such as cooking, shopping, and community mobility. There are now a number of separate 'transitional living units' that specialize in this area. They are often funded from medico-legal assessments and there are a few available on the NHS in the UK. Such units will also teach a wide range of social skills, such as skills at initiating and carrying on a conversation, retaining friends, finding appropriate social outlets, interests, and hobbies, etc.

Vocational rehabilitation

Regrettably it is common for brain-injured people not to return to work, or if they do return to work then lose their job because of the whole range of cognitive, behavioural, and emotional problems that often develop. There is evidence from the USA that a 'job coach' system improves the chance of finding and retaining work. The job coach is a skilled vocational counsellor who will work with the brain-injured person and slowly reintroduce them to the work environment. They will work alongside the person on the job helping them to adapt not only to the work itself but to the necessary social and interpersonal skills that go with the job. This will help to educate and train colleagues as well as more senior managers and employers. One study doubled the employment rate after the introduction of such a scheme.

There are a few vocational rehabilitation units in the UK but mainly in the private sector and once again funded out of damages from a legal settlement. There is a growing demand for such services to reduce the individual's dependence on disability benefits. Joint working across health, social care and voluntary agencies is resulting in support for return to work for people with a variety of issues including traumatic brain injury.

Case management

In the later stages the involvement of a wide range of health, social service, and employment professionals is often needed. Access and coordination of these different professionals can be a major problem for the disabled person and their family. It is becoming increasingly common for a case manager to be appointed who can assist with such coordination and who can often act as an advocate for the disabled person and their family. For some, contact need only be in the short term, but for many people after severe brain injury life-long support is needed from the case manager and many members of the rehabilitation team.

Further reading

1. Wood RL and McMillan TM (ed.) (2001). *Neurobehavioural disability and social handicap following traumatic brain injury.* Psychology Press, East Sussex, UK
2. Ponsford J, Sloan S, and Snow P (1995). *Traumatic Brain Injury. Rehabilitation for everyday adaptive living.* Lawrence Erlbaum & Associates, London
3. Seeley HM and Hutchinson PJ (2006). Rehabilitation following traumatic brain injury: challenges and opportunities. *Advances in Clinical Neuroscience & Rehabilitation,* **6**(2). Available online at http://www.acnr.co.uk/pdfs/volume6issue2/v6i2management.pdf

Spinal cord injury

Background

Spinal cord injury is an excellent example of the improvement in survival and quality of life that can follow from a modern rehabilitation programme. In the early part of the twentieth century nine out of ten people with spinal cord injury died within 1 year and only 1% survived in the long term. Now life expectancy is only modestly reduced. A 20-year-old male would normally be expected to have around 58 years of further life and this is reduced to about 48 years in those with paraplegia and in those with tetraplegia to around 35 years of further life.

- Annual incidence of spinal cord injury is around 10–15 cases per million per annum.
- Mean age of injury is 33 years and the mode 19 years.
- Most injuries occur in males (around 82%).
- The commonest cause is road traffic accidents (40%) but with an increasing proportion from violence and a significant proportion from domestic and industrial falls and sporting injuries.

The incidence of road traffic injuries is reducing secondary to seat-belt legislation, traffic calming measures, and car safety devices.

Early acute management

At the roadside it is important to avoid unnecessary worsening of the spinal cord injury. Individuals should be immobilized in a semi-rigid collar and the individual—if other injuries allow—should be placed in a lateral position with the head kept in line with the spine by the underlying arm. Transportation should be on a spinal board with the head immobilized. Speed of evacuation is important and individuals should be transferred as soon as possible to a regional spinal injuries unit (other life-threatening injuries may need treatment before transfer).

The level of spinal injury cannot be determined solely by examination. There may be some bruising, tenderness, or deformity but there may be no clue as to the exact nature and extent of the underlying injury. Radiographic investigation of high standard is critical. CT and/or MRI scanning may also often be necessary.

Initial management of injuries to the cervical spine would usually consist of skeletal traction applied through skull callipers. This will help stabilize and splint the spine. The standard initial treatment for thoracic and lumbar injuries is simple support in the correct posture usually with a pillow under the lumbar spine to maintain the normal lordosis.

It is very controversial whether conservative management is sufficient or whether operative fixation of the damaged spine produces better results. Around 60% of people in the USA undergo spinal surgery but the incidence in the UK and other parts of Western Europe is much lower. In the UK surgical intervention is reserved for those with unstable displaced fractures and conservative management is the normal practice for stable and undisplaced fractures.

Some centres use a short course of high-dose methylprednisolone in the early stages, started within at least 8 hours of injury. This may improve eventual outcome. This practice is not standardized across UK spinal injury units as there is not sufficient evidence for its use.

Dermatomes, myotomes, and associated reflexes

These are summarized in Fig. 20.1.

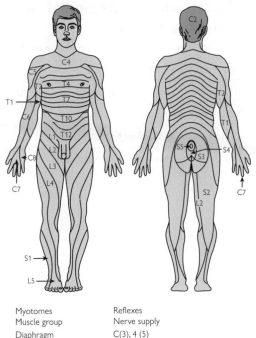

Myotomes	Reflexes	
Muscle group	Nerve supply	
Diaphragm	C(3), 4 (5)	
Shoulder abductors	C5	
Elbow flexors	C5, 6	Biceps jerk C5, 6
Supinators/pronators	C6	Supinator jerk C6
Wrist extensors	C6	
Wrist flexors	C7	
Elbow extensors	C7	Triceps jerk C7
Finger extensors	C7	
Finger flexors	C8	
Intrinsic hard muscles	T1	Abdominal reflex T8-12
Hip flexors	L1, 2	
Hip adductors	L2, 3	
Knee extensors	L3, 4	Knee jerk L3, 4
Anide dorsiflexors	L4, 5	
Toe extensors	L5	
Knee flexors	L4, 5 S1	
Ankle plantar flexors	S1,2	Ankle jerk S1, 2
Toe flexors	S1,2	
Anal sphincter	S2, 3, 4	Bulbocavernosus reflex S3, 4
		Anal reflex S5
		Plantar reflex

Fig. 20.1 An *aide mémoire to* examination—summary of the dermatomes, myotomes, and associated reflexes

General post-acute management— management of the spine

Most people will be managed conservatively. However, one advantage of considering surgery is that the individual can be mobilized more quickly. If a conservative approach is adopted, mobilization is more difficult in the first few weeks. Cervical spine traction is usually maintained for around 6 weeks and at this point individuals must be carefully monitored to make sure there are no respiratory problems and pressure sores are avoided. Once the fracture site is stable the individual can be sat up in bed and normally a halo brace can be used instead of skull traction. This allows early mobilization. The halo brace is kept on for 10–12 weeks until the site is properly stable. In thoraco-lumbar injuries the period of bed rest will usually be 8–12 weeks followed by bracing and gradual mobilization.

General post-acute management— management of medical problems

In the early stages careful monitoring needs to take place to avoid unnecessary medical complications. These mainly consist of:

Respiratory problems

Respiratory insufficiency can occur in people with cervical cord injuries as the intercostal muscles can be paralysed and in high cervical lesions the diaphragm can also be paralysed. Respiratory function can decline quite quickly and careful monitoring needs to be maintained. Regular chest physiotherapy is vital. Pulmonary embolism is also a risk and anti-coagulation is usually advised.

Pressure sores

There is a high risk of pressure sores. Individuals will need to be nursed on a pressure-relieving mattress and their position regularly changed. The skin must be kept clean. Pressure sores are nearly always preventable. If they occur they can be very slow to heal and sometimes plastic surgery is required. Septicaemia from pressure sores is still one of the leading causes of death with spinal injury.

Bladder problems

In the period of spinal shock the bladder is usually non-contractile so that catheterization may be appropriate. Once spinal shock has worn off the commonest problem is detrusor hyper-reflexia giving rise to frequent passage of small quantities of urine associated with urgency. Detrusor sphincter dyssynergia and detrusor hypo-reflexia are also possible, the latter tending to occur when there is damage to the sacral nerves. The management of bladder difficulties is outlined in Chapter 7 (💭 see Bladder detrusor-sphincter dyssynergia, p.112; Management of urinary problems, p.114).

Bowel management

In the period of spinal shock the bowel remains flaccid and should not be allowed to over-distend. Manual evacuation is usually needed. Later bowel evacuation can usually be triggered by glycerin suppository or by anal digital stimulation. Advice on a good-quality high-fibre diet is necessary in the longer term.

Spasticity and contractures

Spasticity can be a major problem in spinal injury. Contractures are nearly always preventable by careful positioning, physiotherapy, and anti-spastic treatment, such as botulinum toxin. The management of spasticity is covered in further detail in Chapter 6.

Heterotopic ossification

This is the development of bone in an abnormal anatomical position in the soft tissues. It is reasonably common in spinal cord injuries, although the prevalence varies between 5–50%. It commonly occurs around hips and knees, causing a decrease in range of movement and sometimes localized swelling, joint effusion, and pain. Treatment is difficult. Etidronate disodium is probably the most useful treatment. Surgical intervention is usually unsatisfactory.

Deep venous thrombosis

This is a significant problem after spinal injury. The wearing of TED stockings and commencement on low molecular weight heparin is advised. Some centres now also use external pneumatic calf compression. Patients with spinal cord injury do not require long term thromboprophylaxis unless there is a history of thromboembolic disease.

Pain and dysaesthesia

Peripheral pain is quite common. Deep burning neuralgic pain can also occur. This is often resistant to treatment but can respond to the use of anti-convulsants and tricyclic anti-depressants. Pain from other sources, such as musculoskeletal causes and osteoarthritis, can also occur.

Autonomic dysreflexia

This is a potentially fatal problem seen in cervical cord injuries above the sympathetic outflow but sometimes in those with high thoracic lesions above T6. It is categorized by:
- Exaggerated autonomic response to a stimulus below the level of the lesion. Such stimuli can include:
  - Distension of the pelvic organs, such as bladder, colon, and rectum.
  - Catheterization.
  - Urinary infections.
  - Sexual intercourse.
  - Pressure sores.
  - Tight clothing.
  - Surgical procedures.

It presents as sudden uncontrolled rise in blood pressure—systolic pressure reaching up to 250–300mm Hg; diastolic pressure 200–220mm Hg.

Other features may include:
- Headaches.
- Sweating.
- Vasodilatation.
- Nasal obstruction.
- Paraesthesia.
- Anxiety.
- Significant hypertension.

Awareness of the problem is important and avoidance of unnecessary stimulation is clearly desirable. Treatment is directed towards reducing blood pressure. Sublingual nifedipine or intravenous hydralazine can be used in more severe cases. Chlorpromazine is another possibility.

Later rehabilitation

Once the individual is mobilizing then rehabilitation can continue at a greater pace. At the point of mobilization it should have become clearer about final functional level of the spinal injury. Initial recovery may have taken place and an accurate functional assessment can be carried out. The level of the lesion clearly has an important bearing on functional outcome (Table 20.1).

Rehabilitation will mainly comprise of intensive physiotherapy and occupational therapy.

Physiotherapy interventions
• Maintenance and improvement of respiratory function.
• Strengthening preserved muscle.
• Stretching programmes to maintain and increase muscle length. This may require serial casting/splinting.
• Spasticity management.
• Bed mobility and transfer techniques.
• Wheelchair skills—self propelling or power wheelchairs.
• Standing practice using tilt tables, standing frames, callipers.
• Gait re-education dependent on the level of the lesion.
• Provision of lower limb orthotics, e.g. callipers, ankle foot orthosis.

Occupational therapy interventions
• Maximizing hand function.
• Splinting.
• Facilitating care tasks and enabling activities of daily living, e.g. dressing practice.
• Provision of aids, equipment, and adaptations to facilitate independent living.
• Community activities.
• Environmental assessment regarding return to home and advice and recommendation on adaptations to property.
• Facilitating return to work.

Nursing interventions
• Skin care.
• Bowel and bladder management.
• Sexual function.

Table 20.1 Expected residual functional ability according to the level of lesion

Level of injury	Complete lesions
Lesion below C3	Dependent on others for all care
	Diaphragm paralysed, needs permanent ventilation or diaphragm pacing
	Chin-, head-, or breath-controlled electric wheelchair
Lesion below C4	Dependent on others for all care
	Can breathe independently using diaphragm
	Can shrug shoulders
	Can use electric wheelchair with chin control
	Can type/use computer with a mouth stick
	Environmental control system operated by shoulder shrug or mouthpiece
Lesion below C5	Can move shoulders and flex elbows
	Can eat with a feeding strap/universal cuff
	Can wash face, comb hair, clean teeth using feeding strap/ universal cuff
	Can write using individually designed splint and wrist support
	Can help in dressing upper half of body
	Can push manual wheelchair short distances on the flat provided that pushing gloves are used with capstan rims on the wheels
	May be able to transfer across level surfaces using sliding board and a helper Electric wheelchair needed for functional mobility
Lesion below C6	Can extend wrists Still needs strap to eat and for self-care
	Can write using individually designed splint but may not need wrist support
	Can dress upper half of body unaided
	Can help in dressing lower half of body
	Can propel wheelchair up gentle slopes
	Can be independent in bed, car, and toilet transfers
	Can drive with hand controls
Lesion below C7	Full wrist movement and some hand function, but no finger flexion or fine hand movements
	Can do all transfers, eat, and dress independently
	Can drive with hand controls
Lesion below C8	All hand muscle s except intrinsics preserved
	Wheelchair independent, but difficulty, but difficulty in going up and down kerbs
	Can drive with hand controls
Lesion below T1	Complete innervation of arms
	Totally independent wheelchair life
	Can drive with hand controls

Walking Index for Spinal Cord Injury (WISCI)[1]

The WISCI scale was developed in 2000[1] initially for use in multi centre trials, however it would be equally valuable as an outcome measure during rehabilitation. See Table 20.2 for the 2001 revision (WISCI II).[2]

Table 20.2 WISCI II[2]

Level	Description
0	Client is unable to stand and/or participate in assisted walking.
1	Ambulates in parallel bars, with braces and physical assistance of two persons, less than 10 metres.
2	Ambulates in parallel bars, with braces and physical assistance of two persons, 10 metres.
3	Ambulates in parallel bars, with braces and physical assistance of one person, 10 metres.
4	Ambulates in parallel bars, no braces and physical assistance of one person, 10 metres.
5	Ambulates in parallel bars, with braces and no physical assistance, 10 metres.
6	Ambulates with walker, with braces and physical assistance of one person, 10 metres.
7	Ambulates with two crutches, with braces and physical assistance of one person, 10 metres.
8	Ambulates with walker, no braces and physical assistance of one person, 10 metres.
9	Ambulates with walker, with braces and no physical assistance, 10 metres.
10	Ambulates with one cane/crutch, with braces and physical assistance of one person, 10 metres.
11	Ambulates with two crutches, no braces and physical assistance of one person, 10 metres.
12	Ambulates with two crutches, with braces and no physical assistance, 10 metres.
13	Ambulates with walker, no braces and no physical assistance, 10 metres.
14	Ambulates with one cane/crutch, no braces and physical assistance of one person, 10 metres.
15	Ambulates with one cane/crutch, with braces and no physical assistance, 10 metres.
16	Ambulates with two crutches, no braces and no physical assistance, 10 metres.
17	Ambulates with no devices, no braces and physical assistance of one person, 10 metres.
18	Ambulates with no devices, with braces and no physical assistance, 10 metres.
19	Ambulates with one cane/crutch, no braces and no physical assistance, 10 metres.
20	Ambulates with no devices, no braces and no physical assistance, 10 metres.

American Spinal Injury Association Impairment Scale (ASIA)

- To gain some form of standardization of classification of injury the ASIA scale[3] (Table 20.3) was developed in the 1990s based upon the original Frankel scale.[4]
- It grades severity of neurological loss and has now been adopted by almost every major organization associated with spinal cord injury.

Table 20.3 ASIA

A	Complete	No motor or sensory function is preserved in the sacral segments S4–S5
B	Incomplete	Sensory but not motor function is preserved below the neurological level and includes sacral segments S4–S5
C	Incomplete	Motor function is preserved below the neurological level and > half of key muscles below the neurological level have a muscle grade of <3
D	Incomplete	Motor function is preserved below the neurological level and > half of key muscles below the neurological level have a muscle grade of >3
E	Normal	Motor and sensory function is normal

References

1. Ditunno Jr JF, Ditunno PL, Graziani V, *et al.* (2000). Walking index for SCI (WISCI) an international multicenter validity and reliability study. *Spinal Cord*, **38**, 234–43.
2. Dittuno PL and Dittuno Jr JF (2001). Walking index for spinal cord injury (WISCI II): scale revision. *Spinal Cord*, **39**, 654–6.
3. American Spinal Injury Association. International standards for neurological classification of spinal cord injury (2000). Revised 2000, Chicago IL: American spinal injury association.
4. Frankel HL, Hancock DO, Hyslop G, *et al.* (1969). The value of postural reduction in the initial management of closed injuries of the spine with paraplegia and tetraplegia *Paraplegia* **7**: 179–192.

Longer-term issues

Discharge home

This is a particularly difficult time. It is better to have a phased discharge with trial home visits. Very commonly houses will need adaptation for a wheelchair and other structural alternations made to improve access—both internal and external. Sometimes hoisting equipment will need to be put into the house and adaptations made to the toilet, bathroom, and kitchen. Environmental control equipment may be needed. There is a need for psychological support over this period of transition both for the injured person and their family. Anxiety and depression are both common at this time. There needs to be smooth transition and a case conference between hospital and community staff is an absolute requirement. Contact with the spinal unit should be maintained and many centres now have outreach workers who can monitor the situation and refer the individual back to the specialist care in the centre as necessary.

Emotional problems

This can be a very anxious time for the injured person as well as family and friends. Clinical depression is common and occurs at some point in at least 50% of spinal-injured people. There is some risk of suicide. Counselling and psychological support is vital and sometimes medication is needed.

Sexual life

Sexual ability depends on the level and completeness of the spinal lesion. Men with complete upper motor neuron lesions will have reflex but not psychogenic erections. Even reflex erections are usually impossible in those with parasympathetic lesions. Satisfactory erection can often be achieved by mechanical means, such as vacuum erection or compressive retainer rings or intracavernosal drugs. However, the introduction of sildenafil is now reducing the need for such mechanical assistance. Orgasm remains possible even in those with complete spinal cord lesions. In women problems can result from lack of vaginal lubrication. Self-image and self-confidence can be severely affected and sexual counselling is often required. Individuals should be counselled about the totality of sexuality as there is a tendency for discussions to focus on penetrative sexual intercourse.

Fertility

Fertility is usually not reduced in women. However, fertility is often reduced in men who have low sperm counts with diminished sperm motility. Sometimes if ejaculation is not possible it can be induced by direct stimulation or by electroejaculation. Fertility can be improved by techniques such as *in vitro* fertilization or intracytoplasmic sperm injection. Women with spinal cord injury may have problems in labour, particularly if the lesion is above T10 and autonomic dysreflexia is a risk. However, this should not necessarily discourage women from becoming pregnant as good quality obstetric care will clearly reduce such risks.

Later medical complications

Pathological fractures

As there is a higher risk of osteoporosis in paralysed limbs then there is an increased risk of pathological fractures.

Post-traumatic syringomyelia

This occurs in about 4% of people and consists of an ascending myelopathy due to secondary cavitation in the central part of the cord. It usually presents with pain in the arm with characteristic disassociated sensory loss—reduced pain and temperature sensation but preservation of proprioception. Motor loss of the lower motor neuron type occurs and a sensory loss can spread to the face (syringobulbia). Surgical treatment includes decompression and drainage of the central cavity.

Respiratory management

Those with high cervical cord lesions who have lost diaphragmatic function require long-term ventilatory support. Modern ventilators can be mounted on a wheelchair. Speech is possible with an uncuffed tracheostomy tube that allows air to escape to the larynx and in some people a phrenic nerve stimulator can achieve diaphragmatic ventilation.

Issues of participation

Leisure pursuits

There are now a wide variety of leisure pursuits possible for those with spinal cord injury. Ideally integration to able-bodied clubs should be encouraged but there are specific clubs for those with spinal injuries, particularly wheelchair sports.

Driving

Driving a motor vehicle in modern society is increasingly vital. Driving should be possible at all levels of spinal injury except perhaps for those with very high cervical cord lesions. Automatic transmission is important and hand controls are usually essential. A variety of infra-red devices to control secondary function, such as windscreen wipers, lights, and horn are available. Very light powered steering makes life easier for those with a weak grip. Individuals with cervical lesions who retain some useful shoulder and upper function can still drive a car using a variety of driving devices attached to the steering wheel. There are a number of devices that can stow a wheelchair safely. Adapted vehicles are now readily available—if expensive—to enable people to drive from their wheelchair. The UK now has a number of specialist driving assessment centres for proper assessment of the necessary adaptations.

Employment

Regrettably only around 25–35% of people with spinal cord injuries return to work. The chances are higher in younger people or those already in a job at the time of injury. Although returning to and retaining a job is not easy individuals should be encouraged to contact the disablement employment advisors who can provide both advice and financial help.

Information

The key to independence is access to good quality information. Individuals should be kept informed of developments at all times and put in touch with the necessary range of professionals, not only health but also in social services, employment, and in other spheres. Much valuable support can be gained from the local spinal injuries association. The internet now provides an excellent source of information and advice and training in computer literacy should be encouraged by the rehabilitation team.

The management of spinal cord injury can pose a range of challenges to the multidisciplinary team. At the present time we cannot yet promote natural recovery but many useful interventions are possible. Individuals with spinal injury can certainly continue to have a good quality of life and many should be able to work and fully participate in society.

Further reading

1. Bromley I (ed.) (1998). *Tetraplegia and Paraplegia: A Guide for Physiotherapists*, 5th edn. Elsevier Science, London.
2. Grundy D and Swain A (ed.) (2002). *ABC of Spinal Cord Injury*. BMJ books, London.
3. Royal College of Physicians (2008). *Chronic spinal cord injury: management of patients in acute hospital settings. Concise Guidance to Good Practice Series, No 9*. Royal College of Physicians, London.
4. ⌐ www.sci-info-pages.com—quadriplegic, paraplegic and caregiver resources.
5. ⌐ www.mascip.co.uk—multidisciplinary association of Spinal Cord Injury Professionals.
6. ⌐ www.spinal.co.uk—Spinal Injuries Association.
7. ⌐ www.aspire.org.uk—supporting people with spinal injuries.
8. ⌐ www.basics.pwp.blueyonder.co.uk—British Association of Spinal Cord Injury Specialists.
9. ⌐ www.iscos.org.uk—International Spinal Cord Society (ISCOS).

Parkinson's disease and movement disorders

Parkinson's disease

In the last 30 years there have been huge improvements in the drug therapy of Parkinson's disease so that in the early stages disability and handicap are kept to a minimum. However, in the later stages there is a less satisfactory response to dopaminergic therapy and major problems of disability and handicap can arise. Thus, Parkinson's disease is still a major rehabilitation challenge, often to the geriatric rehabilitation team.

Causes of parkinsonism

It is important to remember that there are many different causes of parkinsonism some of which need specific treatment in their own right (e.g. Wilson's disease). Table 21.1 outlines some of the causes of parkinsonism.

The importance of awareness of the different causes of parkinsonism is not only that some need different treatments but that others respond much less well to standard dopaminergic therapy. Progressive supranuclear palsy and various multiple system atrophies, for example, do not respond at all well to therapeutic intervention and symptom management becomes the mainstay of rehabilitation.

Epidemiology

Parkinson's disease is by the far most common cause of parkinsonism. The prevalence is around 150–200 per 100 000 population in the UK and an incidence of 18–20 per 100 000 population per annum. The male:female ratio is around 3:2. The disorder becomes much more common with increasing age, and approximately 1 in 10 people over the age of 80 will have parkinsonism of various causes. However, the mean age of onset is 55 years and so it is not exclusively a problem of the older population and can occur in people who are still economically active.

Table 21.1 Causes of parkinsonism

Class of disorder	Manifestation
Degenerative diseases	Parkinson's diseasev
	Progressive supra-nuclear palsy
	Multiple system atrophies
	Olivopontocerebellar atrophy
Infections	Post encephalitic parkinsonism
Drug or toxin induced	Neuroleptics
	Carbon monoxide poisoning
	Manganese poisoning
	MPTP-induced parkinsonism
Vascular conditions	Cerebrovascular disease
	Hypertensive encephalopathy
Trauma	Head injury
	Punch drunk syndrome
Cerebral tumour	Alzheimer's disease
Other neurological conditions that may have parkinsonian features	Intermittently raised pressure hydrocephalus
	Various forms of Huntington's disease
	Wilson's disease

MPTP, methyl-4-phenyl-1,2,3,6-tetrahydropyridine.

Principal features

There are three main features of Parkinson's disease:

- Hypokinesis or reduced movement, including:
  - Delay in initiation.
  - Poverty of movement.
  - Imprecision.
  - Slowness of movement—bradykinesia.
  - Fatigue.
  - Problems with automatically associated movements—such as arm swing and reduction of facial expression.
- Rigidity:
  - Increased resistance to passive muscle stretch throughout the range of movement—lead pipe.
  - Rigidity is usually present in the trunk as well as the limb muscles.
  - Rigidity is responsible for the stooped posture characteristic of the disease.
- Tremor:
  - Is usually a slow coarse rest tremor and is often more of an embarrassment than a functional problem.
  - It is usually the hypokinesia and rigidity that cause the main functional difficulties.

The other component is *impaired postural reflexes*. The individual pushed from in front tends to stagger backwards or pushed from behind tend to stumble forwards. This disequilibrium is often reflected in everyday difficulties such as maintaining balance in a crowded environment or when trying to hurry or change direction.

Medical management

The details of medical management are the subject of neurological textbooks. However, as the medical management is the mainstay of treatment in Parkinson's disease some relevant points can be made.

The key to treatment of Parkinson's disease is direct replacement of levodopa which needs to be combined with carbidopa (a peripheral decarboxylase inhibitor) that reduces peripheral side effects. There are now many combinations of carbidopa/levodopa as well as various controlled-release forms. Drugs come in different formats, such as tablets or liquids. It is often a matter of trial and error to find the right balance of appropriate dopa replacement therapy. In general terms it is usually best to give smaller doses at frequent intervals throughout the day. Obviously the minimum dose compatible with the desired reduction in symptom levels is necessary. This should mean that treatment varies according to the handicap of the individual. Treatment is usually more aggressive in a younger person who is still at work and needs a reasonable degree of control and coordination—sometimes at the expense of side effects. In the older person who simply needs to get around the house adequately then a less aggressive treatment is necessary. In the older person side effects are usually more problematic.

Some authorities would start treatment as soon as the diagnosis is made, while others would wait as late as possible so that the complications of treatment are delayed. There is still no clear consensus on this issue. However, most people would now start treatment as and when symptoms become troublesome and interfere with daily life. Once again this usually means early intervention for the young active person and later intervention for disabled elderly people. The general treatments now available are:

- Dopa replacement therapy—co-careldopa or co-beneldopa in various formats.
- Dopamine agonist agents, such as bromocriptine, pergolide, lysuride, cabergoline, ropinirole or pramipexole—some are now available as transdermal patches (rotigotine).
- Dopamine B-oxidase inhibitors—selegiline, thought to slow progression of disease until more recent studies have thrown some doubts on long-term efficacy and safety. Rasagiline is another example.
- Catechol-O-methyltransferase (COMT) inhibitors—these drugs prolong the effect of carbidopa/levodopa therapy by blocking an enzyme that breaks down dopamine. Tolcapone and entacapone are examples.
- Anticholinergic drugs can be useful in milder cases although troublesome side effects include confusion, dry mouth, blurred vision, constipation, and impaired erection.
- Self-injected apomorphine (direct acting D_1 dopamine agonist with rapid onset of action) can be useful when there are late-stage complications and 'rescue' is required from a bad rigid period.
- The medical management of Parkinson's disease is now increasingly complicated with a wide range of potential agents. It is not appropriate in this textbook to list the dose schedules of the various medication regimens and reference should be made to standard Parkinson's textbooks as well as detailed information from the drug manufacturers.

Any form of dopamine replacement therapy is usually very effective for several years. However, after 5–10 years of treatment difficulties can begin to arise. The person can begin to swing from a rigid phase ('off') to a phase of marked dyskinetic movements ('on'). This on/off swinging can be manifest in a variety of patterns, and the dosage and timing of treatment becomes increasingly difficult. At this point the input of a specialist neurological Parkinson's disease service becomes necessary.

There has recently been renewed interest in stereotactic neurosurgical procedures, usually deep stimulation of three target areas—the thalamus, subthalamic nucleus, and globus pallidus. There has also been recent interest in implantation or neural grafting techniques to boost cerebral dopamine production but such techniques are neither widely proven nor widely available.

In recent years the discovery of gene mutations for familiar or inherited forms of Parkinson's disease has led to a significant increase in research on Parkinson's disease genes and the function of proteins that are encoded by those genes. Thus, further identification of gene defects may help not only to understand Parkinson's disease but perhaps offer treatment, at least for some sub-groups, in the future. Currently identified genes include *alpha-synuclein, Parkin, DJ-1, pink-1, DRDN* and others. Gene therapy certainly may be a future potential treatment as may be the administration of neurotrophic or neuroprotective agents. A useful up-to-date website is providing by the National Institute of Neurological Disorders and Stroke.[1]

References

1. http://www.ninds.nih.gov/disorders/parkinsons_disease/parkinsons_disease.htm

Rating scales

Accurate clinical assessment is a fundamental part of rehabilitation medicine and assessment in Parkinson's disease is no exception. As usual, individual symptoms should have their own measures but it is sometimes useful to have an overall disability rating scale. There are a few that have been validated for Parkinson's disease. The commonest are the staging scales of Hoehn and Yahr and the disease rating scales of Webster (Tables 21.2 and 21.3). There are other more comprehensive tools, such as the Unified Parkinson's Disease Rating Scale,[1] that are mainly used for research purposes.

Table 21.2 Standard scales in Parkinson's disease—staging*

Stage	Description
I	Unilateral involvement, little or no functional impairment
II	Bilateral or midline involvement without impaired balance
III	First signs of impaired writing reflexes; some functional restriction but capable of independent living and may be able to work
IV	Fully developed severe disabling disease; can stand and walk unaided
V	Confined to wheelchair or bed

*After Hoehn MM and Yahr MD (1967). Parkinsonism: onset, progression and mortality. *Neurology*, **17**, 427–42.

Table 21.3 Standard scales in Parkinson's disease: disease rating.*
A clinical rating (0–3) is given for each of the 10 items with 0 = no involvement and 3 = severe (instructions being given for each)

Item	
1	Bradykinesia of hands—including handwriting and pronation–supination
2	Rigidity—proximal and distal
3	Posture—head flexion, 'poker' spine, and simian posture
4	Upper extremity swing
5	Gait—stride length, shuffling
6	Tremor—amplitude and constancy
7	Facies—mobility
8	Seborrhoea
9	Speech
10	Self-care

*After Webster DD (1968). Critical analysis of the disability in Parkinson's disease. *Modern Treatment*, **5**, 257–82.

References

1. http://www.mdvu.org/library/ratingscales/pd/

Treatment of symptoms in Parkinson's disease

Gait

The most obvious problem in Parkinson's disease is the shuffling and unsafe gait which can cause frequent falls. Bradykinesia and rigidity are the problems largely responsible, combined with impaired postural reflexes. The gait problems can also be made worse by dyskinetic movements as a result of treatment.

There is now evidence that a physiotherapist can definitely improve gait, although the exact type and duration of therapy is not really known. It is probable that a home-based physiotherapy programme is useful and is certainly the most appreciated by the individual.

The physiotherapist can teach various trick strategies that can overcome some of the problems. Some examples are:
- Freezing—in this phenomenon the individual suddenly freezes as if the feet were stuck to the floor. This can be helped by getting the person to pretend that they have to step over a small obstruction. Freezing in a chair can be helped by being taught to gently rock backwards and forwards until there is sufficient momentum to rise.
- The slow and shuffling gait can be improved by auditory cues.
- Severe and painful rigidity can be helped by simple stretching exercises.
- There seems to be some value (probably psychological and social as well as physical) in group therapy sessions.

It is important that physiotherapy contact is maintained throughout the illness. Short bursts of physiotherapy for further training and advice is probably the best methodology available when there are scarce resources. The physiotherapist will often have to work in conjunction with the neurologist or geriatrician so that the drug therapy can be manipulated in order to maximize mobility at the most relevant times of day for that individual.

Activities of daily living

The same problems of bradykinesia, rigidity, and tremor will often cause problems with fine hand and arm movements. Involvement by the occupational therapist and other team members can make real improvements. There is now a large variety of suitable aids that can assist including:
- Large-handled cutlery.
- Plate guards.
- Use of Velcro® instead of buttons.
- Writing aids.
- Various home-based assessments in order to maximize functional use in the kitchen, bedroom, bathroom, etc.

Speech and swallowing problems

Communication can become difficult in parkinsonism. The speech is characteristically described as dysarthrophonic—a combination of problems of articulation and phonation. It is usually a monotonous pitch combined with a quiet voice with words coming in short rushes at variable rates due to the impaired breath control. Stuttering can also occur. Referral to a speech therapist is useful at the earliest possible stage. Appropriate speech exercises can produce significant improvements in intonation, stress, and rhythm and in more advanced stages various forms of augmentative communication aid can be prescribed.

Regrettably the problem of coordination also affects swallowing. The assessment of swallowing is described in Chapter 9 (see Swallowing, p.134). The involvement of a speech therapist, dietician, and radiographer is essential. Dietary manipulation may be needed, and accurate diagnosis rests on videofluoroscopy. There are various speech techniques that can improve swallowing, although most emphasis is usually placed on appropriate changes in food consistency whilst maintaining adequate nutritional intake.

Autonomic problems

Problems with bladder function occur in around 50% of people with Parkinson's disease and are probably secondary to autonomic dysfunction which occurs as part of the disease process. The commonest symptoms are:

- Frequency.
- Urgency.
- Urge incontinence.
- Sometimes hesitancy and retention.

The situation can be complicated and urodynamic evaluation is often necessary. Other problems of autonomic function can also occur. The commonest is *postural hypotension* often leading to fainting on getting out of bed or getting up from a seat. This occurs more commonly in some of the other parkinsonian syndromes, particularly the Shy–Drager syndrome and other Parkinson plus syndromes. Treatment is difficult but can include:

- Advice on avoiding rapid changes of posture.
- Avoiding large meals.
- Avoiding excessive alcohol.
- Avoiding warm temperatures.
- Avoiding excessive straining.
- Use of compressive garments, such as elastic stockings or abdominal binders (often impractical).
- Treatment with fludrocortisone.

Constipation is also common, although drugs, particularly anticholinergic drugs, might be responsible. Dietary manipulation can be helpful as well as adopting a regular pattern of defecation. Laxatives and other bulk forming agents should be avoided if at all possible but can be helpful in resistant cases.

Pain

It is usually thought that sensory symptoms are not present in Parkinson's disease and sensory signs are absent. However, it is quite common for cramp-like pains and diffuse aches and pains to be present. In an older population such difficulties can of course be secondary to musculoskeletal problems, such as a result of osteoarthritis. Sometimes pain can go hand in hand with the short-term disease fluctuations, such as the on/off swinging, which can be helped by appropriate drug manipulation.

Sleep disorders

Disorders of sleep are very common in Parkinson's disease. The commonest is sleep fragmentation characterized by recurrent waking which may in turn be due to the inability to turn over at night because of the bradykinesia and rigidity. Daytime fatigue is consequently common. Drug manipulation might be needed in order to try to get an appropriate dopaminergic effect overnight. There are now various devices that can help someone turn over in bed. These vary from the very simple—such as a strap attached to the bed head—or the even simpler device of wearing cotton socks which gives some purchase on the sheets. There are now also automatic beds that will tip slightly helping the individual turn over.

Sexual function

It is likely that the autonomic dysfunction in Parkinson's disease can also result in problems of erection in the male. In addition both sexes can be troubled by mechanical problems during sex secondary to the physical impairments. The situation is often compounded by drug effects, particularly anticholinergics which can dry secretions and cause erectile problems. The involvement of a sexual counsellor is useful. Sexual problems can often be helped by:
• Simple advice on timing of drugs.
• Advice on posture.
• Counselling to deal with problems of self-image and relationship difficulties.
• Alternative means of sexual stimulation.

Cognitive and emotional problems

Depression is very common in Parkinson's disease and occurs in >50% of the parkinsonian population at some point during the disease. As in many neurological problems there is a tendency to assume that depression is a natural accompaniment of the disorder and for it not to be treated adequately. There is no evidence that depression in the context of Parkinson's disease responds any worse than depression in other contexts and it should be treated just as aggressively (☐ see Treatment of depression, p.204).

Clinical anxiety can also be a problem but is normally a result of inadequate information, advice, and counselling.

Dementia is undoubtedly more common in Parkinson's disease and the incidence is around 20–30%. It is obviously more common in other forms of parkinsonism and indeed parkinsonism can be associated with

Alzheimer's disease itself. Dementia in the context of Parkinson's disease is often characterized by:
- Increasing dependency.
- Increasing indecision.
- Increasing passivity.
- Memory problems.
- Perseveration.
- Slowness of thought.
- Problems with new learning.
- Increasing 'mental' inflexibility.

It is often the dementia that causes increasing family stress and involvement of psychogeriatric services can be needed in the later stages.

Issues in service delivery

The preceding sections have shown that there is a wide range of problems in Parkinson's disease requiring input from a whole multidisciplinary team. In the case of Parkinson's disease the team should undoubtedly have medical input, usually from a neurologist or geriatrician with a particular interest in Parkinson's. There are now a number of hospital or community-based Parkinson's teams providing long-term contact, help, and advice. As with all chronic neurological problems, accurate information, advice, and counselling, not only to the affected person but also to the family, is vital at all stages.

Individuals should be put in contact with local Parkinson's disease or other relevant societies, which can provide useful literature written in lay terms. Fortunately in the UK there has been the development of specialist nurses specifically trained in the management of Parkinson's disease. Such nurse practitioners can provide invaluable help, advice, and support, including advice on drug manipulation. This reduces the amount of time the individual may need to spend in neurological or geriatric outpatient clinics. The nurse practitioner could be the main point of contact for access to the whole variety of health and social services.

Further reading

1. Edwards M, Quinn N, and Bhatia K (2008). *Parkinson's disease and other movement disorders.* Oxford University Press, Oxford.
2. ⊕ www.ninds.nih.gov/disorders/parkinsons_disease/parkinsons_disease.htm
3. ⊕ www.nlm.nih.gov/medlineplus/parkinsonsdisease.html—a useful and comprehensive website with links to a variety of other information resources for Parkinson's disease.
4. ⊕ www.parkinsons.org.uk—the UK Parkinson's Disease Society. This website is highly recommended particularly for people with Parkinson's disease and their carers.
5. ⊕ www.cochrane.org/reviews—there are now >100 Cochrane reviews of different aspects of Parkinson's disease and parkinsonism treatment. A very useful resource for up-to-date systematic reviews of the subject.

Dystonia

Dystonia is defined as a sustained involuntary muscle contraction involving abnormal movements and postures. There are many types of presentation and some of the commoner sites are as follows:

- Neck—spasmodic torticollis or cervical dystonia.
- Eye—blepharospasm.
- Jaw, tongue, and mouth—oromandibular dystonia.
- Larynx and vocal cords—spasmodic dysphonia.
- Arm and hand muscles—various segmental, multifocal, and hemidystonic forms.
- Generalized dystonia—usually but not invariably starting in childhood.

In addition there are various occupational cramps which usually, but not always, occur in the context of an occupation with repetitive movements, such as writer's cramp or various musician's cramps or sportsman cramps, such as dystonia of the hand muscles occurring in professional darts players.

The dystonias are uncommon but not rare. A recent survey showed a prevalence of around 26 per 100 000 population for all types of dystonia.

Aetiology is normally unknown, although there is emerging evidence of a genetic predisposition and now at least 20 genetic disorders are described in specific dystonic families. It is likely that dystonia has a genetic predisposition but requires an environmental trigger—which is usually unknown. Occasionally dystonia can be symptomatic of another process and a thorough neurological examination and, if necessary, investigation is needed. Hemidystonia, for example, can follow stroke or traumatic brain injury or be a manifestation of underlying brain tumour.

Important secondary causes are drug-induced dystonias, caused by the psychotrophic medications for example.

Treatment

In a few cases specific treatment is required—such as in Wilson's disease. Occasionally surgical removal of tumours or arteriovenous malformations might be needed. However, in the vast majority of cases such specific measures are not possible. The treatment of choice for the focal dystonias is now undoubtedly *botulinum toxin*. Botulinum toxin acts by blocking the transmission of acetylcholine at nerve endings and thus weakening the appropriate muscles. The toxin is delivered by intramuscular injection and takes 2–3 days to take effect. The effect then lasts around 3 months before new nerve endings sprout and the injection needs repeating. The injection is remarkably safe and the only real problem is a flu-like illness occurring in about 1% of those injected. Sometimes there can be difficulties of over-weakening the injected muscles, such as dysphagia as a complication of injection for spasmodic torticollis.

In a few people (around 3–5%) the injection does not work or there is later non-response probably due to the formation of antibodies. In such cases the use of oral drug therapy may still be necessary.

The prescription of the right drug can be time-consuming. Overall around 40% of people find a drug that suits their dystonia but about half of these individuals have unacceptable side-effects. Thus, only about one in five people will eventually find a drug that is appropriate and helpful. The drugs that can be used are:

- Anticholinergics.
- Muscle relaxants—baclofen.
- Benzodiazepines such as clonazepam.
- Dopamine agonists (there is a rare form of dystonia that responds immediately and extremely well to dopamine but the other forms of dystonia can sometimes respond reasonably well).
- Dopamine antagonists.

Sometimes surgical procedures can be useful. There are various procedures for specific focal dystonias. These include:

- Surgery to lift the eyelids in blepharospasm.
- Surgery on the neck muscles for spasmodic torticollis.
- Various forms of brain ablative or stimulation procedures, particularly for hemidystonias.

Other therapy

As dystonia is such an unusual condition it is important that good-quality literature is given for information, help, and advice. The Dystonia Society produces excellent and readable literature in the UK. Depression and anxiety can occur and access to a counsellor can be helpful. There is some evidence that complementary medicine, such as hypnotherapy and acupuncture, can help in certain resistant cases. Various members of the multidisciplinary team may need to be called upon for advice, such as the speech therapist for dysphonia, or the full team may be needed for the more widespread generalized dystonias.

Further reading

1. Edwards M, Quinn N, and Bhatia K (2008). *Parkinson's disease and other movement disorders.* Oxford University Press, Oxford.
2. ⍈ www.dystonia.org.uk—the website of the UK Dystonia Society which provides an excellent web resource for those with dystonia and their families.
3. ⍈ www.wemove.org—an excellent general website for dystonia and a wide variety of other movement disorders. Mainly orientated to the non-health professional but nevertheless provides a very useful resource for any member of the multidisciplinary team involved in movement disorders. The website also contains slide sets on movement disorders.

Huntington's disease

Huntington's disease is a rare condition with a prevalence of only around 2–10 per 100 000 population. It is a degenerative disorder in which neuronal loss occurs in the caudate nucleus and putamen with a characteristic finding of atrophy in the head of the caudate nucleus on MRI scanning.

Genetics

Huntington's disease is an autosomal dominant condition with virtually full penetrance so that each offspring of an affected parent has a 1 in 2 risk of inheriting the disorder. The gene (*Huntingtin*) has now been mapped (to the tip of the short arm of chromosome 4) and the responsible gene was identified in 1993. A diagnostic test is now available with a very high sensitivity and specificity—virtually 100%. Genetic counselling is key to management in this disorder as pre-symptomatic testing is now possible. There are now useful protocols for the management of pre-symptomatic testing and such testing should be carried out only in recognized centres. The protocol typically includes:

- One or two sessions on the general features and inheritance of Huntington's disease.
- The next few sessions concentrate on the issues of pre-symptomatic testing and a blood sample is taken if the client wishes to go ahead.
- One pre-test session is initially arranged with a psychiatrist to reduce the risk of severe psychiatric reaction following the test.
- A session where the result is given on a face to face basis.
- Appropriate follow-up arrangements, particularly counselling, both after a positive result and after a negative result. Contact should be made soon after the result either by telephone or a home visit.

The peak age of onset is around 40 years, which obviously means that the person is often married with a young family and thus with a high risk of having passed on the genetic defect to the offspring. Onset can rarely occur before the age of 20 and rarely after 60. Onset is insidious but time from diagnosis to death is around 10–15 years. There is a characteristic spectrum of motor, psychiatric, and cognitive problems.

Motor features

Involuntary movements, particularly chorea, are seen in most, but not all, people. Facial chorea is particularly common. Gait can be unsteady and dyspraxic. Dysarthria can occur and swallowing can be compromised. Sometimes other involuntary movements are present, such as dystonia. Apraxia can also occur when testing the arm.

Psychiatric disorders

Psychiatric problems are virtually universal. Often there are insidious changes in personality and behaviour that pre-date the first physical symptoms. Apathy can be present but a more common pattern is irritability with outbursts of verbal and physical aggression. Sometimes an individual will go on to more overt psychiatric illness including major depression or even schizophrenia-like manifestations. Euphoria and manic episodes have also been reported.

Cognitive impairment

There is a wide range of cognitive problems even in the early stages of Huntington's disease. Subtle intellectual decline can even be detected in carriers of the genetic mutation before any symptoms are present. Speech can be halting with long pauses and there are often problems with word finding and naming difficulties. Writing can be impaired, but fortunately reading is usually reasonably well preserved. Many people report difficulty in planning, requiring considerable support and assistance from their family and carers. Visuospatial tasks can be affected, which adds to the overall dementing illness. Obviously memory problems can be particularly difficult as frank dementia progresses.

Treatment and support

Huntington's disease is not curable but a rehabilitation team can provide invaluable assistance and support:

- Physiotherapy can improve gait and reduce unnecessary physical complications, such as contractures.
- Occupational therapy can assist with activities of daily living and planning of the home and work environment.
- Speech and language therapy can be used for the management of dysphagia and communication problems.
- A dietician can be useful as there is often a significant increase in calorific requirements in someone with constant movements.
- A neuropsychological or neuropsychiatric assessment is essential as depression, behavioural problems, and dementia begin to take effect.

A dedicated team managing people with Huntington's disease in each region provides the best quality service, assistance, and support to the Huntington's population.

Further reading

1. Edwards M, Quinn N, and Bhatia K (2008). *Parkinson's disease and other movement disorders*. Oxford University Press, Oxford—this up-to-date Oxford Specialist Handbook on Parkinson's disease and other movement disorders also provides an excellent chapter on Huntington's disease.
2. www.hda.org.uk—the UK Huntington's Disease Association, which is the standard website for those with the disorder and their families as well as providing good quality background information for health care professionals.
3. www.wemove.org—an excellent general website.
4. www.nlm.nih.gov/medlineplus/huntingtonsdisease.html—also provides an excellent information resource which is more geared towards health professionals.
5. www.ninds.nih.gov/disorders/huntington/huntington.htm— Huntington's disease information page from the National Institute of Neurological Disorders and Stroke.

Motor neuron diseases

Background

Motor neuron disease (MND) is characterized by progressive degeneration of motor neurons:

- Anterior horn cells–resulting in lower motor neuron lesions.
- Cortico spinal tracts—resulting in upper motor neuron lesions.
- Motor nuclei in brain stem—resulting in both upper and lower motor neuron lesions.

Sensory lesions are rare and cranial nerves affecting sight and lower sacral segments of the spinal cord affecting continence are spared.

The MNDs usually have a progressive course leading to death within 3–5 years of diagnosis. However, there can be considerable rehabilitation potential in terms of reducing the risk of unnecessary complications and promoting quality of life. This is particularly important as people nearly always retain normal cognitive function and full conscious appreciation of their disability. It is the role of the rehabilitation team to help the individual and their family overcome the feeling of powerlessness.

Textbooks of neurology should be referred to for a detailed discussion of classification, pathology, aetiology, and diagnosis. However, there are a few points that should be mentioned which are of relevance to the rehabilitation team.

Motor neuron diseases

It is important to remember that although adult-onset MND accounts for around 90% of cases there is an increasingly important range of other MNDs and it is very likely that over the next few years further genetic disorders will be identified which may eventually lead to different treatment possibilities. The following is an abbreviated classification of MNDs as currently understood.

- *Amyotrophic lateral sclerosis (ALS)*— most common, affects 65%. Mixture of upper and lower motor neuron problems giving rise to characteristic signs including spasticity, increased reflexes, and muscle weakness in combination with muscle wasting and muscle fasciculation.
- *Progressive bulbar palsy*—a form of ALS which affects 25%. A similar combination of lower and upper motor neuron problems but mainly involving the bulbar muscles giving rise to additional problems such as dribbling, dysarthria, dysphagia, and respiratory difficulties.
- *Progressive muscular atrophy*—affects <10%. Only affecting the lower motor neurons of the limbs with a better survival.
- *Primary lateral sclerosis*—affects approximately 2%. A rarer form only involving upper motor neurons.
- *Sporadic MND* —so called as for 95% of cases the disease develops for no apparent reason. Current research suggests that this may develop as a result of a combination of genetic susceptibility and lifestyle and environmental factors.
- Familial MND— accounts for around 5% of all MNDs and an increasing number (currently around 20%) have an identified genetic locus. Currently 20% have a mutation in chromosome 21 involving copper/zinc superoxide dismutase. Clinically the sporadic and familial forms are indistinguishable. There are other rarer genetic and inherited forms of MND.

- Western Pacific amyotrophic lateral sclerosis/parkinsonism/dementia complex.
- Juvenile onset MND—with intracytoplasmic conclusions.
- MNDs with definable causes:
  - Post-polio syndrome.
  - Heavy metal intoxication.
  - Hexosaminidase-A deficiency.

The precise diagnosis is obviously important and is likely to become increasingly important as more genetic and biochemical abnormalities are determined.

Epidemiology

The prevalence of MND is around 5 per 100 000 population with an incidence of around 1–2 per 100 000 population per annum. There are areas of geographical concentration where the incidence exceeds 100 times the average (including the western Pacific island of Guam, several specific villages in Japan, and the Irian Jaya region of Papua New Guinea).

MND is mainly a disease of late middle age, with an age of onset in the 50s and 60s. There are a greater number of males than females, with a ratio of approximately 3:2. The average duration of symptoms to death is around 2–3 years with survival a little longer in younger patients and those with progressive muscular atrophy.

Diagnosis

The symptoms of presentation can vary enormously. Motor weakness and the absence of sensory loss is probably the most common presenting feature, although sometimes the first complaint can be of muscle cramps or fasciculations or muscle wasting. Diagnosis still rests largely on clinical history and examination often supported by neurophysiological evidence of denervation in the muscles of at least two limbs.

No diagnostic tests exist but neurological investigations should normally include EMG, nerve conduction tests, blood tests, and may also include MRI, lumbar puncture, myelogram, muscle biopsy, and CT to exclude other possibilities.

Giving the diagnosis

The diagnosis of MND is usually fairly straightforward in the majority of cases. It is said that around 80% of people can be diagnosed within a few minutes, 10% need some further investigations to exclude other pathologies, and in 10% of people the diagnosis only becomes apparent after several months of symptom progression. Thus, in the majority of people an accurate diagnosis can be given quite quickly. Obviously imparting the diagnosis is a particularly anxious time for the patient and family. Boxes 22.1 and 22.2 give standards of care recommended by the MND association.[1]

Box 22.1 At diagnosis—sensitive communication of the diagnosis, ensuring:[2]

- Appropriate emotional/psychological support.
- Appropriate information made available, in a timely manner, about:
  - The condition and its implications.
  - Sources of help and support.
  - The MND association and national helpline.
- Comprehensive information sent to the GP.
- Follow-up clinical appointment within 2 weeks of diagnosis.
- Direct referral to MND Association Regional Care Adviser (RCA).

Box 22.2 Following diagnosis—immediate identification of a single point of contact (keyworker) to ensure:[2]

- Access to information and service provision.
- Planning and co-ordination of support and care.

Although needs will vary according to the individual, the following elements are essential:
- Access to information, service provision, and benefits tailored to current needs of person about MND.
- Informed holistic approach to assessments.
- Flexibility and priority of response to ensure speed in service delivery.
- Access to appropriate expertise and services at the appropriate time, including:
  - Specialist palliative care and respite care.
  - Speech and language therapy.
  - Physiotherapy.
  - Occupational therapy.
  - Dietetics.
  - Social care.
  - Gp/primary health care team.
  - Neurology and neurorehabilitation.
  - Respiratory specialist.
  - Psychologist.
- Access to pharmaceutical and other relevant treatments.
- Regular communication between disciplines.
- Regular monitoring and review.
- Continual offer of association support:
  - Helpline.
  - RCA.
  - Branch.

References

1. www.mndassociation.org
2. Reproduced from www.mndassociation.org

Treatment and rehabilitation

Medical treatment

Regrettably, at the time of writing, there is no single agent that is confirmed to slow down disease progression. Many promising therapies have not stood the test of larger-scale double-blind, placebo-controlled studies. The most promising treatment focuses on anti-glutamate therapy and riluzole, a sodium channel blocker that inhibits glutamate release, seems to be the most promising such agent. Two large-scale studies have demonstrated a modest benefit and prolonged survival in MND. Other large-scale studies are under way both with other anti-glutamate agents and with several neurotrophic factors. The results of these studies are still awaited.

Rehabilitation management

Mobility and activities of daily living

The main aims of intervention for the physiotherapist are to maintain mobility muscle strength and joint mobility preventing joint stiffness and pain. Most people will relatively quickly progress to wheelchair dependency and then an appropriate wheelchair and seating needs to be prescribed with proper cushioning to reduce the risk of pressure sores.

The occupational therapist will work with the patient to enable them to maintain independence for as long as possible through provision of assistive devices and equipment, ranging from jar openers and mobile arm supports to bath lifts.

There is a variety of simple aids to daily living which can produce significant functional benefit and the input of both physiotherapy and occupational therapy is important for a functional assessment and treatment regime to be put into place.

Respiratory and bulbar problems

One of the most distressing difficulties arises from bulbar involvement. The following symptoms can occur:

- Dysphagia arises from muscle weakness and problems of coordination of the tongue and swallowing mechanism. An assessment by a speech and language therapist is required, often involving videofluoroscopy and the involvement of a radiographer and dietician (📖 see Examination of swallowing, p.130).
- Feeding can often become slow and tiring and it may be preferable to use a percutaneous endoscopic gastrostomy (PEG) feeding regimen sooner rather than later. This will maintain calorific intake, reduce the length of time spent on feeding, and reduce, but not entirely remove, the risk of aspiration, pneumonia, and malnutrition.
- Dribbling can be a particular difficulty. Anti-cholinergic drugs or patches can be helpful but can be associated with troublesome side-effects, particularly constipation, dry mouth, and urinary problems. Recently, injection of the salivary glands with botulinum toxin has been shown to be useful for this troublesome symptom.

- Dysarthria and communication problems—advice from a speech and language therapist is invaluable. At the end stage, short-term loan of assistive communication devices can often be helpful to maintain quality of life and the ability to communicate not only with family and friends but also strangers.
- Respiratory failure—involvement of the respiratory muscles of the neck and intercostals as well as phrenic nerve damage can all seriously compromise respiration. Physiotherapy input is important at this point for advice and treatment regarding chest drainage, intermittent suction, and positioning. Portable suction devices should be available within the home. There may come a point when ventilatory assistance is required. At this stage ethical dilemmas are not uncommon and judgements sometimes need to be made after broad discussion with the individual, family, and the rehabilitation team as to whether quality of life would be improved in the short term by artificial ventilation or whether such measures would uncomfortably prolong life. Non-invasive intermittent positive pressure ventilation via a mask is the most practical form of assistive ventilation. The equipment is portable and can be used on a wheelchair. Ventilatory support during sleep can lead to subjective improvement in sleep and resolution of morning headaches and reduction of fatigability during the daytime. 24-hour intermittent positive pressure ventilation via a tracheostomy tube is only rarely used. Antibiotics would normally be given for chest infection unless pneumonia is overwhelming. For severe anxiety or panic a small dose of lorazepam sublingually can be helpful. If breathlessness causes distress during the later stages of the disease then small amounts of morphine can be useful, even though it is a respiratory depressant.

Other features

Pain is not usually present in the early stages of MND but is quite common in the later stages and is often due to musculoskeletal problems in combination with muscle cramps, spasticity, and other factors such as constipation. Treatment obviously depends on the cause but non-steroidal anti-inflammatory agents can be useful to ease the musculoskeletal aches and pains.

Emotional problems

Almost all people with MND will go through a period of clinical anxiety and depression. Hopefully such problems need not become severe if proper support is given and counselling is available. As usual lack of knowledge goes hand in hand with unnecessary anxiety. Psychological and psychiatric support should be available as necessary. A few people have the troublesome problem of emotionalism, including pathological tearfulness and laughter, probably because of bulbar involvement. Small doses of anti-depressants can significantly help such symptoms.

Terminal care

Most studies show that people prefer to stay at home during their terminal stage. This will often require complex, albeit short-term, care packages involving experienced nurses with the support of the rehabilitation team. Death is usually from bronchopneumonia. Small doses of morphine and/or prochlorperazine and hyoscine can be used to relieve distress and diminish bronchial secretion.

In many countries ethical questions are now arising with regard to assisted suicide. In virtually all countries this remains illegal. However, it should be pointed out that no physician has an ethical, legal, or moral obligation to prolong the distress of a dying individual. Post-bereavement counselling should also be available to the family who have often gone through a very traumatic period.

Service delivery

The preceding sections clearly demonstrate that MND requires the complex interaction of a variety of health professionals. There is little doubt that individuals with MND are best managed by a comprehensive multidisciplinary rehabilitation team. The team should be available to offer specialist advice at all times and regular reviews should be offered in case unrecognized complications are beginning to arise. The advent of MND specialist nurses is a useful development, and such people can often act as the key point of contact with the rest of the team. There are now a number of examples of MND specialist teams around the UK and abroad. Such teams often have access to a wide range of equipment and assistive technology devices—including environment control equipment and communication aids—that can be loaned in the short term.

Further reading

1. Williams AC (ed.) (1994). *Motor Neuron Disease*. Chapman & Hall Medical, London.
2. www.mndassociation.org/—website of the Motor Neuron Disease Association.

Disorders of the peripheral nerves

Background

Accurate diagnosis is important for the rehabilitation of people with disorders of the peripheral nerves. There are a small but increasing number of disorders that are now specifically treatable. Even in those disorders of peripheral nerves that do not currently have a specific treatment accurate diagnosis remains important in order to determine natural history and prognosis. This will help to determine the rehabilitation strategy. Some conditions are spontaneously recoverable—such as Guillain–Barré syndrome—whilst others are progressive—such as the hereditary motor and sensory neuropathies. Some may require surgical intervention, e.g. the brachial plexus injuries. This section will cover the following disorders of peripheral nerves in order to indicate the range and extent of rehabilitation techniques:

- Critical illness polyneuropathy.
- Guillain–Barré syndrome.
- Post-polio syndrome.
- Hereditary motor and sensory neuropathies.
- Brachial plexus injuries.

Disorders of peripheral nerves usually consist, in varying proportions, of the following problems:

- Weakness—lower motor neuron weakness, particularly affecting the arms and legs.
- Variable degrees of sensory disturbance.
- Troublesome pain, either directly as a result of the peripheral nerve damage or secondary to abnormal gait and posture.
- Retained intellect.

Nerve conduction studies, electromyography (EMG) and sometimes *nerve biopsy* may all be necessary not only to determine the diagnosis but to determine the prognosis. There may, for example, be evidence of complete denervation (poor prognosis), partial denervation (better prognosis) or some denervation with evidence of re-innervation (good prognosis).

The rest of this chapter will deal with different types of peripheral nerve disorders from acute, severe, and reversible conditions to chronic and steadily progressive problems.

Further reading

1. Mendell JR, Kissel JT, and Cornblath DR (2001). *Diagnosis and Management of Peripheral Nerve Disorders.* Oxford University Press, Oxford.

Weakness

Virtually all peripheral nerve lesions are associated with weakness, and from a functional point of view weakness affecting the arms and legs is the most disabling. In acute polyneuropathies (e.g. Guillain–Barré syndrome) weakness of the trunk muscles and respiratory muscles can clearly have a more immediate detrimental effect as respiration may be depressed. In other forms of peripheral nerve disorders there can be difficulties with swallowing or head control which brings additional rehabilitation challenges.

Weakness can cause the following problems:
- Reduced walking ability secondary to weak leg muscles.
- Easy tripping over rough ground or even carpets.
- Reduced functional ability in the arms.
- Contractures—it is usually thought that contractures are only associated with upper motor neuron spasticity but contractures of the soft tissues are not uncommon if the effects of gravity are not counteracted by appropriate splinting in individuals with lower motor neuron problems.

The following may be needed:
- Passive movements of the limbs—particularly in the acute phase—should prevent contractures.
- Splinting can restore function, particularly in the arm.
- Provision of an ankle–foot orthosis can correct weak dorsiflexion, improve gait, and prevent falls.
- Exercise can improve muscle strength, although it probably does not improve the rate of recovery of the underlying neuropathy. Isometric and isotonic exercises both increase muscle power and exercise tolerance but there is little information on the precise amount of such exercise required for maximum effect.
- People with longer-term weakness may need adaptations to their immediate environment, such as ramps, lifts, wheelchairs, special utensils, and other hand adaptations (e.g. pen holder, etc).
- Other home and work adaptations, such as environmental control equipment, can also help to reduce the disability associated with chronic arm and leg weakness.

Sensory disturbance and pain

Loss of normal sensation carries a significant risk of unnoticed trauma with the consequent dangers of *neuropathic ulceration* and *neuropathic arthropathy*. Individuals must be taught to be aware of the problem and examine areas of abnormal sensation regularly. They should be very careful with the use of appropriate footwear and expert *chiropody* is essential for those with sensory disturbance in the feet.

Involvement of sensory nerves can lead to severe *neuropathic pain*. Neuropathic pain is variously described but words often used are constant, deep, and burning. The treatment of neuropathic pain can be very difficult but may include:

- Anti-convulsants—particularly carbamazepine, gabapentin and pregabalin.
- Tricyclic anti-depressants—such as amitriptyline.
- SSRI antidepressants—such as venlafaxine.
- Tramadol.
- Cannabis or cannabinoids.
- Local or regional sympathetic blockade.
- Use of a TENS machine.

It is also important to remember that in some people an abnormal gait or posture can lead to secondary musculoskeletal pain. Involvement of a physiotherapist is vital in order to normalize gait as much as possible as well as provide appropriate seating and postural support. The most useful drugs for musculoskeletal pain are the non-steroidal anti-inflammatory agents.

Other problems can arise and will need treatment in their own right:

- Pressure sores—📖 see p.156.
- Scoliosis.
- Contractures.
- Respiratory depression—📖 see Guillain–Barré syndrome, p.372.
- Poor nutrition, often secondary to feeding problems.
- Depression and emotional disturbance (📖 see p.202), secondary not only to the physical disability but to associated chronic pain.

Guillain–Barré syndrome and critical illness polyneuropathy

Guillain–Barré syndrome

Guillain–Barré syndrome is rare and only affects between 1–2 people per 100 000 population per year. The key features are:

- Often rapid onset usually in a matter of days but sometimes a matter of hours.
- Advancing weakness often starting in the feet but rapidly moving upwards to involve the muscles around the knees and hips and then the hands, wrists, elbows, and shoulders.
- Around 20% of people develop respiratory weakness requiring artificial ventilation.
- Can also be associated with bulbar weakness and autonomic failure.
- Treatment involves plasmapheresis and/or intravenous IgG infusion as soon as possible after the start of the illness.
- Prognosis is reasonable but a significant minority will remain disabled in the long term. A recent study showed that around 60% make a complete recovery. However, 8% die in the acute phase, 4% remain ventilator dependent, around 10% are unable to walk unaided, and the remainder have some residual physical disability.
- Prognosis is difficult to predict but older people, those unable to walk within 4 days of onset or those requiring artificial ventilation tend to have a poor outcome.
- Acute management focuses on the need to monitor respiratory function and start ventilation as necessary. Acute management will also require careful monitoring of positioning to minimize the risk of contractures and pressures.
- Urinary and chest infections are a particular risk in the early stages.
- Autonomic dysfunction can result in severe postural hypotension.
- Recovery can be slow and require a considerable amount of rehabilitation.
- Fatigue can be a real difficulty in the recovery phase.
- Depression is common.
- Support from ex-patients can be useful and, in the UK there is a national Guillain–Barré support group.[1]

Critical illness polyneuropathy

This is a relatively newly recognized problem first described in 1984. It usually consists of severe axonal peripheral neuropathy arising in the context of people admitted to intensive care with severe sepsis and/or multiple trauma. In one study about half of individuals on intensive care for >7 days had documented evidence of peripheral neuropathy. The key points are:

- Recognize the syndrome.
- Ensure proper limb posture in order to minimize the risk of pressure sores and limb contractures.
- Use orthoses as necessary to maintain limbs in a neutral position.

- Rehabilitation usually follows the same lines as Guillain–Barré syndrome.
- Usually there is a good prognosis although recovery can take many weeks.
- A small proportion has long-term disability and thus will need long-term support.

References

1. ⭧ www.gbs.org.uk—the website of the Guillain–Barré syndrome support group, provides up-to-date information as well as professional links.

Post-polio syndrome

Acute polio is now rare and has virtually been eradicated in the developed world and is significantly less common in developing countries. However, there are still a large number of people who were affected by the disease, usually in their childhood. It is now increasingly recognized that late deterioration after polio can occur. The key points are:

- Post-polio syndrome usually occurs around 30–40 years after the acute illness.
- It is defined as the development of new neuromuscular symptoms (e.g. fatigue, muscle joint pain, weakness, increasing muscle wasting, etc.).
- It arises in the context of post-polio with no other determined cause.
- Sometimes the resulting disability can be disproportionate to the apparent minor change because of lack of functional reserve in people who are already disabled.
- Deterioration is usually slowly progressive. It is said that, on average, there is about 1% of loss of muscle strength each year. However, even a modest reduction in muscle strength of, say, 10% can be enough to produce severe further weakness in individuals already disabled after their acute polio.
- Fatigue can be a major symptom.
- Muscle pain, particularly cramping pain after exercise, can also be common.
- Aerobic training can improve muscle strength, at least to a limited degree.
- Treatment will focus on methods to assist weak limbs, such as the use of orthoses, mobility aids, wheelchairs, and environmental adaptation.

Further reading

1. ⌂ www.britishpolio.org.uk—a large UK charity supporting people with polio and the post-polio syndrome.
2. Jubelt B (2004). Post-polio syndrome. *Current Treatment Options in Neurology*, **6**, 87-93—an up-to-date summary.
3. Howard RS (2005). Polio myelitis and the post-polio syndrome. *British Medical Journal*, **330**, 1314–18—a further up-to-date summary.
4. Farbu E, Gilhus NE, Barnes MP, *et al.* (2006). EFNS guideline on diagnosis and management of post-polio syndrome. Report of an EFNS Task Force. *European Journal of Neurology*, **13**, 795-801—a comprehensive guideline and literature summary.

Hereditary motor and sensory neuropathies

There is an increasing genetic literature on a variety of hereditary motor and sensory neuropathies (HMSN). Slowly a number of genetic defects are being described, and it is quite likely in future years that some of these conditions will be treatable. However, at the moment there are no cures available for any form of HMSN. Rehabilitation will centre on:

- Proper diagnosis.
- Information and explanation regarding the nature of the condition.
- Description of the natural history so that appropriate future provisions can be made both by the treating rehabilitation team and the person and family.
- Possibility of genetic counselling for other members of the family.
- Physiotherapy advice regarding maintenance of a maximum degree of muscle strength.
- Appropriate prescription of orthoses and footwear to minimize the risks associated with soft tissue contracture.
- Regular chiropody is particularly important for those with sensory loss in the feet and hands.
- Provision of appropriate hand splints and other simple aids to daily living, such as adapted cutlery, pen holders, etc.
- Prescription of mobility aids, such as walking frames and wheelchairs and appropriate advice about driving and transport.
- Adaptation of the environment as necessary, such as ramps, lifts, hoists, assistive technology, etc.
- Surgical correction is sometimes necessary. This can involve Achilles tendon lengthening, plantar fasciotomy, posterior tibialis, long flexor and extensor tendon transfers, as well as the possibility of arthrodesis and osteotomies in order to preserve function and prevent complications.
- Progression is generally slow. Unnecessary complications should not be allowed to arise.

Finally, it should not be forgotten that some forms of peripheral neuropathy are quite treatable. This would include diabetic neuropathy where tight control of the diabetes is important. Rarer forms of neuropathies, such as vitamin B_{12} deficiency or vitamin E deficiency, can improve dramatically with appropriate replacement therapy. The reader is referred to neurological texts for a definitive list of the causes of peripheral neuropathy and for a more detailed discussion of the various genetic forms of HMSN.

Further reading

1. ⌘ www.charcot-marie-tooth.org—the USA Charcot–Marie–Tooth association for people with Charcot– Marie–Tooth and other neuropathies.
2. ⌘ www.ninds.nih.gov/disorders/neuropathy_hereditary—a good summary of up-to-date research and further links to the various sub-types of hereditary neuropathies and Charcot–Marie–Tooth disorders from the National Institute of Neurological Disorders and Stroke in the USA.
3. Goodman BP and Boon AJ (2008). Critical illness neuromyopathy. *Physical Medicine and Rehabilitation Clinics of North America*, **19**, 97–110—a very up-to-date review of the subject.

Brachial plexus injuries

Brachial plexus injuries are uncommon but nevertheless around 500 people in the UK suffer permanent disability each year—usually from traction injuries to the plexus. Brachial plexus injuries in childbirth still occur but they are becoming less common as obstetric practice improves. Road traffic accidents account for the great majority and indeed most are secondary to motorcycle accidents. The mean age is in the early 20s and the majority are males.

Individuals should be referred as soon as possible to a specialist centre where there is not only a good multidisciplinary rehabilitation team but also where expert surgical advice and treatment is obtainable.

Treatment will focus on:
• A very accurate diagnosis of the parts of the brachial plexus that have been damaged. This will involve a careful functional assessment often combined with neurophysiological investigation.
• If rupture or avulsion of the spinal nerves is suspected then surgical exploration should be carried out as soon as possible. There is a clear decline in long-term functional results if surgery is delayed. One series showed full return of function in individuals who were operated on within 3 weeks of the injury. However, the proportion of failures rose to over 60% in those operated on after 6 months. The nerves can be repaired either by grafting or nerve transfers.
• Specialist splints can be very useful and effectively restore function in individuals who do not make a full recovery after surgery. The following are particularly helpful:
  • An elbow lock splint is useful in the absence of active elbow control (C5 and C6 lesions).
  • A gauntlet splint is useful when there is major loss of function in the forearm and hand (C7, C8, and T1 lesions).
  • The flail arm splint is used when there is irreparable damage to the whole plexus (C5–T1 lesions). The flail arm splint will include an elbow hinge and a wrist platform to which can be attached various devices, such as split hook which is open and closed by a cable and operated from the opposite shoulder. Various other appliances can be attached to the flail arm device, such as attachments to aid activities of daily living around the house or in the garden. Some individuals can return to work using various splints attachments, such as pliers, sewing devices etc.

In summary the outlook is good for people with brachial plexus lesions as long as urgent referral is made to a specialist centre and the lesion is surgically explored and repaired as soon as possible. There is often much that can be done for those with residual arm and shoulder weakness. However, often the main disabling feature in the longer term is the presence of central neuropathic pain. This can be difficult to control. Treatment will focus on the use of anti-convulsants and/or tricyclic anti-depressants.

Further reading

1. Gilbert A (ed.)(2001). *Brachial plexus injuries.* (Federation of European Societies for Surgery of the Hand). Martin Dunitz, London— a definitive textbook on the subject but summarizing the disorders and treatment from a surgical perspective.
2. ᵺwww.ubpn.org—there are surprisingly few brachial plexus patient groups, this is the United Brachial Plexus Network based in the USA.
3. ᵺwww.brachialplexuspalsyfoundation.org—a further USA-based website.

Epilepsy

Background

Epilepsy is common. Around 1% of the entire population will suffer at least one non-febrile seizure during their lives. The overall prevalence is around 5000 per 100 000 population with an incidence of around 50 per 100 000 population per annum. It is the most common disabling neurological condition in both adults and children. It is not a condition that is often seen by a multidisciplinary rehabilitation team. Epilepsy is intermittent and normally people function perfectly well in between fits without any associated disability. The management of epilepsy is normally restricted to a neurological service supported by specialist regional centres. Around the UK there are three residential establishments for people with persistent and intractable epilepsy.

Medical management

This section will specifically not deal with the classification of epilepsy or with the details of pharmacological anti-convulsant management. These are outside the remit of this book. However, some points can be made:

- Accurate diagnosis is essential. Diagnosis and investigation needs to rule out causes of secondary epilepsy which may lead to other potential treatments. Causes would include brain tumour, cerebrovascular disease, and a whole variety of inherited metabolic problems. Accurate diagnosis may obviously help prediction with natural history and prognosis and guide potential treatment.
- Accurate description of the type of epilepsy is important in order that appropriate anti-convulsant medication can be initiated if required.
- The great majority of individuals (>80%) can be quite well controlled on a single anticonvulsant. Only a small minority will need combination anti-convulsant medication and such individuals need to be seen and monitored in a specialist centre.
- The most commonly prescribed anti-convulsants remain the well-established drugs, particularly carbamazepine, sodium valproate and phenytoin. Generally the newer drugs, such as gabapentin, vigabatrin, topiramate, lamotrigine, etc., are generally used as second-line treatment although some are now beginning to find a place as first-line options. On a global scale phenobarbital is still used because it is cheap and effective, albeit with a very unsatisfactory range of side-effects. Monitoring of serum levels of anti-convulsants can be helpful to determine compliance and to maximize treatment, although not all anti-convulsants can be meaningfully measured in this way. The saturation kinetics of phenytoin need to be borne in mind as increases above, roughly, 300mg daily can lead to dramatic increases in serum levels and consequent toxicity.
- It is important that individuals with epilepsy have long-term follow-up. Seizure type and frequency can change and there is a need for on-going monitoring of anti-convulsant efficacy and side-effects. Only around 6% of the UK epileptic population attend an epilepsy clinic. There is

evidence that such people retain more information about their epilepsy and are more satisfied with the service and support. A dedicated epilepsy service has a number of advantages, including:

- Expert management of the anti-convulsant regimen.
- High-quality support from nursing staff who may be specifically trained in the management of epilepsy.
- Access to expert advice on such matters as driving, employment, etc.
- Psychological and counselling support.
- Support from local epilepsy groups.

Neuropsychological assessment and support

Most people with epilepsy have well-controlled seizures with no significant cognitive problems. However, some, particularly those with frequent or poorly controlled seizures, are at risk of cognitive and intellectual problems. This can be a result of the epilepsy itself, the underlying cause, or as a consequence of anti-convulsant medication.

The commonest difficulties are:
• Memory problems, particularly recent memory.
• Problems with information-processing speed.
• Problems with concentration or fatigue.
• Clinical anxiety and/or depression.

These neuropsychological problems need to be properly assessed and monitored and coping strategies put into place under the guidance of a clinical neuropsychologist. Psychologists can also be helpful in managing anxiety and depression, although sometimes medical input is required. Such symptoms can in themselves trigger seizures which in turn can lead to increased anxiety and thus more seizures, etc. Relaxation therapy can produce a significant reduction in seizure frequency in people prone to clinical anxiety.

Depression is probably best managed by cognitive strategies rather than anti-depressants as the latter can aggravate epilepsy.

Rarely, individuals with complex partial seizures can exhibit aggression during a seizure and the nature of the problem needs to be recognized and such seizures controlled as well as possible. Such individuals can often get into serious problems with the judicial system as a result of epileptic violence.

Social aspects of epilepsy

There are serious difficulties associated with the diagnosis of epilepsy, and there is often a profound effect on social, family, and work life.

Employment

Individuals with epilepsy are at a significantly higher risk of being unemployed compared with the general population. However, there is evidence that a trained epilepsy worker, such as a social worker or nurse, supporting the individual through job applications and interviews and visiting the employer can produce real benefit in terms of increased employment and retention rates. Advice needs to be given on occupations that are clearly inappropriate, such as flying, commercial diving, operating hazardous machinery, working at heights, and driving public service vehicles and commercial driving.

Driving

It is important for the epilepsy team to be fully acquainted with the complex area of driving legislation for people with epilepsy. This will vary from country to country. Driving is an essential part of modern society and an inability to drive can have a very significant impact on employment and social life. It can be vital for people living in rural situations. Inappropriate advice can lead to unnecessary disadvantage. At the present time in the UK people are allowed to drive as long as they have been seizure free for at least 1 year or attacks have only occurred whilst asleep for a period of at least 3 years. However, regulations change and the epilepsy team should be able to give full up-to-date advice from the Driving Vehicle Licensing Agency (DVLA) in Swansea.[1] Responsibility for informing the DVLA falls with the licence holder and not the physician or the epilepsy team. However, the team do have an obligation to society as a whole to inform the DLVA if an individual is known to be driving and is thought to be a significant danger to society through, for example, frequent uncontrolled seizures.

Family

The family of the person with epilepsy needs to be involved in the whole process of diagnosis and on-going treatment. Support and guidance particularly need to be given to children. Such information could include:
- Full discussion about the nature of epilepsy.
- Knowledge of trigger factors, such as tiredness, alcohol, photosensitive triggers, etc.
- A good knowledge of appropriate first aid management during and immediately after a seizure.
- Full discussion on the broader social issues, such as social life, work, and driving.

Families with young children with epilepsy often have a difficult task in balancing normal risk-taking behaviour in children on the one hand and over-protection resulting in potential psychological problems and family strife on the other hand. Involvement of the whole family in appropriate counselling/support is essential.

Overall there is far more to epilepsy than management of anti-convulsant drugs. There is a clear need to involve an expert team in order to minimize disability and promote participation in society.

References

1. ◌ www.dvla.gov.uk/medical.aspx—this is the UK website for the Driver and Vehicle Licensing Agency which provides information on up-to-date driving regulations for those with epilepsy and for other neurological disorders.

Further reading

1. Shorvon S (2005). *Handbook of Epilepsy Treatment*, 2nd edn. Blackwell Publishing, Oxford—a comprehensive and modern guide to all treatment aspects of epilepsy including surgical treatment.
2. ◌ www.epilepsynse.org.uk—website of the National Society for Epilepsy in the UK which is a comprehensive site for people with epilepsy and their families and provides useful background information for health professionals.
3. ◌ www.cochrane.org—there are now over 470 Cochrane reviews on different aspects of epilepsy. The Cochrane review website provides a full list of this ever complicated subject. Recent reviews, for example, include the role of a ketogenic diet and the value of psychological treatments for epilepsy as well as a large number of reviews of specific anticonvulsant drugs.

Dementia

General guidelines

Dementia usually falls within the province of the psychogeriatric team. However, dementia is not that uncommon in the younger population and is associated with a number of common neurologically disabling diseases, including:

- Parkinson's disease.
- Stroke.
- Multiple sclerosis.

There is also some tentative evidence that individuals with traumatic brain injury have a slightly higher risk of dementia in later life. Thus, the multidisciplinary rehabilitation team needs to be familiar with the approaches that can help the person with dementia.

Dementia is defined as a global impairment of function, including:

- Intellectual function.
- Memory.
- Higher perception.
- Language.
- Emotional and behavioural control.

An individual can function quite well in some domains whilst functioning very poorly in others. Thus, the first task is a full multidisciplinary assessment that will enable that particular person's strengths and weaknesses to be identified. Reassessment at frequent intervals is important as dementia is usually a progressive process and areas of initially preserved function can decline over time and different strategies may need to be adopted.

Most people with dementia are looked after in the community by friends and relatives and any rehabilitation process designed to support the person with dementia also needs to support their main carers. The carers must be involved in the assessment process, in designing appropriate strategies, and must be given long-term support. Many people with dementia can continue to live in the community and avoid the indignity and other problems associated with residential and nursing home care. However, others cannot be looked after by carers at home and will need residential admission. The staff in any residential environment obviously must be entirely familiar with the various strategies that can improve the lives of those with a dementing illness.

Rehabilitation in dementia is under-researched and many treatment approaches have not been properly evaluated. However, the next section outlines approaches that have shown to be helpful.

Helpful approaches

Environmental adaptation

People with dementia generally function better in a stable and familiar environment. This is often why people with dementia do quite well at home and, at least initially, do poorly if moved into a residential or nursing home. The physical environment is important and residential settings or rehabilitation units should do what they can to achieve a home-like atmosphere with a domestic style of furniture. People should have their own clothes and possessions in their immediate vicinity. Clear directions and signposting should be available. If individuals are less able to read then colour coding is often useful. For example, blue doors could mean bathrooms and red doors toilets. Basically as much effort as possible should be put into making the immediate environment familiar, routine, and non-threatening.

Stimulation activity

It seems clear that absence of sensory stimulation in some residential environments can compound behavioural disturbance. Some homes are characterized by drab colours, mass-produced furniture, and endless similar corridors. Attempts should be made to personalize the individual's own room as well as the home in general. However, in addition to this commonsense approach there is some, albeit limited, evidence that sensory stimulation including music, touch, taste, and smell can produce short-term benefit. Sensory stimulation can provide carers with some means of interaction. Some physical activity, within the confines of often frail people, and general occupation of time is useful. For example, it is important for the carers to be aware of the individual's previous lifestyle, hobbies, and interests and some attempt should be made to continue to interact with them by continuing with or discussing such interests.

Reminiscence

In dementia, at least in the early stages, individuals' past memories are usually reasonably intact. Thus, the use of a person's own past material, such as photo albums or newspaper cuttings and magazines, can act as prompts and triggers for memory. This can lead to an improved social interaction and probably reduces the risk of unnecessary depression, anxiety, and behavioural disturbance.

Reality orientation

Reality orientation (RO) aims to help the person with dementia continue to experience success and achievement as well as having an increased awareness of present reality. Regular RO sessions up to five times a week lasting about half an hour have shown to be beneficial in terms of orientation. Sessions will often be composed of a small group meeting on a regular basis and working on activities geared to increasing awareness of the immediate surroundings and of people around them. Informal RO will involve the staff and carers on a 24-hour basis keeping the person in touch with current reality, such as the weather, day of the week, current news items, etc. Basically RO helps the person with dementia to continue to experience success and achievement and increase their awareness of present reality. There is evidence that many people with dementia are still able to learn and retain material under the right conditions. For example, a person can be successfully taught a number of face/name associations using prompting techniques that seek to avoid the occurrence of any errors. The absence of errors seems to improve learning.

Drug management

It is known that in people with Alzheimer's disease there is a deficit in cholinergic neurotransmission. The most useful approach seems to involve agents that inhibit the breakdown of acetylcholine by the enzyme acetyl cholinesterase resulting in an increase in the amount of acetylcholine available. Donepezil hydrochloride and rivastigmine are the first of the acetyl cholinesterase (ACE) inhibitors to be licensed for use in Alzheimer's disease. Another licensed drug also includes galantamine. A recent Cochrane review has confirmed the efficacy of these three drugs in terms of improvement in cognitive function in those with mild-to-moderate Alzheimer's disease.[1] There is, so far, no evidence of the differences between them with respect to efficacy. It is possible that donepezil has fewer side effects that rivastigmine but good quality comparative trials are few. Although the long-term impact of the drugs is yet to be established, it does seem clear that these drugs, and newer ones on the market, can apparently slow the progression of dementia, at least in some people with mild-to-moderate cognitive impairment.

In general terms psychotropic drugs should be avoided for the control of behaviour. However, occasionally marked symptoms of excitement, agitation, hallucination, or hostility can be responsive to neuroleptics. Side effects can be a particular concern in the elderly population.

Sleep problems can be very troublesome, particularly for the family. Additional activity in the daytime can be useful by reducing the amount of daytime sleep and by establishment of a calming routine nearer bedtime. Sometimes a modest dose of a hypnotic, such as a benzodiazepine, may be necessary but once again should be avoided if at all possible. It should be remembered that older people do not actually need longer periods of sleep. If, in a nursing home, an individual is put to bed at 8.00pm then it is not surprising that some individuals will then wake at 4.00am after 8 hours sleep!

Behavioural management

Behavioural management techniques have already been described (📖 see p.192). There is some evidence that appropriate behavioural management can produce some benefit for the demented person. Contingent reinforcement techniques in some residential environments have been shown to increase participation in daily activities and mobility as well as improvements in dressing and self-care tasks. Careful assessment of the individual based on the ABC principles (📖 see p.190) can sometimes lead to improvements in inappropriate behaviours and certainly seem worth trying as long as all the staff and/or the family are involved in the process.

Thus, there are a number of strategies which may well improve the lives of people with dementia and whilst not necessarily affecting the dementing process can certainly maximize quality of life both for the demented person and, as importantly, their family and carers.

References

1. Birks J (2006). Cholinesterase inhibitors for Alzheimer's disease. *Cochrane Database of Systematic Reviews*, Issue 1, Article No. CD005593.

Further reading

1. Waite J, Harwood R, Morton I, *et al.* (2008). *Dementia care: a practical manual*. Oxford University Press, Oxford—this provides a good background to dementia care for all members of the multidisciplinary team.
2. Ballard C, O'Brien J, James I, *et al.* (2001). *Dementia: management of behavioural and psychological symptoms*. Oxford University Press, Oxford—this has now become the standard textbook on the management of behavioural and psychological problems in the context of dementia. It is geared towards a medical readership but provides a thorough resume of the subject of relevance to all professional groups involved in the management of people with dementia.
3. ⬦ www.alzheimers.org.uk—the UK Alzheimer's society which provides good web based support for people with Alzheimer's and their carers.
4. ⬦ www.nlm.nih.gov/medlineplus/dementia.html—another excellent website with a wide range of links to many dementia related topics, including research and symptom management.

Chapter 26

Musculoskeletal pain in common rheumatological conditions

Background

>80% of the population will consult a general practitioner for musculoskeletal pain. Most musculoskeletal pain will settle within 3–6 months but in those people whose pain continues to be troublesome, and by virtue of duration becomes chronic their will be two key attributes:

• The pain affects physical, psychological, and social function.
• The individual is not able to carry out their normal activities.

This chapter will focus on some of the main rheumatological conditions that have pain as a central feature as well as impacting on physical function. Each condition will be introduced to the reader along with presenting clinical signs and advice on management. The chapter will commence with a definition of pain and a basic introduction to pain mechanisms.

Definition

The most widely used definition of pain is from the International Association for the Society of Pain which regards pain as 'an unpleasant sensory and emotional experience associated with actual or potential tissue damage or described in terms of such damage'. See Box 26.1.

Pain mechanisms

- In the 17th century pain was seen as purely a physical phenomenon with a direct relationship between the amount of damage or 'nociception' and the pain experienced. What this theory did not explain was the variation in the pain experience for a given stimulus or injury (why do some patients take longer to recover from whiplash than others?) or the persistence of pain beyond the time of tissue healing.
- In 1965 Melzack and Wall[1] revolutionized our understanding of pain mechanisms with the gate control theory of pain. This theory demonstrated that the transmission of pain messages could be modulated within the spinal cord via descending messages from the brain (our cognitions and emotions) or altered by activating another source of sensory receptor (exercise to release endorphins).

Pain receptors

Pain receptors are situated in the tissues especially the skin, synovium of joints and arterial walls. These receptors are activated by various stimuli including:

- Mechanical changes—e.g. excess weight of a particular area.
- Temperature changes.
- Inflammatory changes—the release of prostaglandin, bradykinin, histamine and serotonin.

The peripheral sensory nerves transmit a signal of pain from the peripheries to the central nervous system to enable identification of the stimulus e.g. pain in the wrist. The alpha-(A) delta fibres (thin and myelinated) transmit the sharp pain of an acute injury and the slower C-fibres (unmyelinated) produce the dull aching pain of a more persistent problem. When these fibres are stimulated the 'pain gate' opens and messages pass to the brain to be perceived as pain. When large fibres become activated (A-beta) they close the 'pain gate'. A-beta fibres transmit the sensation of touch, consequently acupuncture and electrical nerve stimulation work on the same principle and excite large fibre activity. Nerve impulses that descend from the brain can also operate 'the gate'.

Box 26.1 The difference between chronic and acute pain

Acute pain is short lived whereas chronic pain is an ongoing experience

Acute pain
Duration is transient
Location usually single site
Identifiable cause

Chronic pain
Duration is persistent
Location is generalized
Often no identifiable cause

References
1. Melzack R and Wall PD (1965). Pain mechanisms: a new theory. *Science*, **150**, 971–9.

Inflammatory arthritis—rheumatoid arthritis

Rheumatoid arthritis (RA) is the most common inflammatory arthritis, with the potential to impact on physical, psychological, and social function. Many patients find it difficult to remain in work and leisure activities are often curtailed. Early diagnosis and treatment is required to try and minimize disability and morbidity. Patients can experience a combination of acute pain, which often occurs when there is a 'flare' of disease activity as well as daily (chronic) pain affecting the muscles and the joints. The frequency of the pain can result in fatigue, low mood, and impinge on functional activities.

Incidence

Population studies suggest an incidence of 3.4 per 10 000 in women and 1.4 per 10 000 in men. Although RA affects all ages, the commonest time of onset in women is in the 3rd–5th decade whilst in men the incidence increases over the age of 45 years.

Cause

The cause is unknown but there is a genetic predisposition that may be triggered by infective, hormonal, or environmental factors. First degree relatives are twice as likely to develop RA than the general population and approximately 50% of patients will carry the antigen HLA DR4.

Diagnosis

Diagnosis is arrived at through a combination of clinical and laboratory tests. Onset is insidious with inflammation, pain, and stiffness present in synovial joints. The metacarpophalangeal, proximal interphalangeal, wrist, and metatarsophalangeal joints are commonly affected with symmetrical changes. Large joint involvement is more common in older patients and often has an acute presentation. Less frequently onset may be characterized by a persistent monoarthritis or oligoarthritis. Laboratory tests and radiographs are used to support the clinical impression of RA and exclude other differential diagnosis. The American College of Rheumatology criteria for the classification of RA is primarily used for research purposes (☐ see Box 26.2).

Laboratory tests results in a patient with active RA

- Raised inflammatory markers—C-reative protein (CRP) and erythrocyte sedimentation rate (ESR).
- Positive immunoglobulin M—rheumatoid factor occurs in 75% of RA patients. It is possible to have RA with a negative rheumatoid factor, where the diagnosis is classified as sero-negative RA.
- Acute phase response including raised gamma GT, alkaline phosphatase and ferritin and a reduction in serum albumin and haemoglobin.

Box 26.2 The American College of Rheumatology criteria for the classification of RA

Four of the following criteria must be present:
- Morning stiffness.
- Arthritis of at least three joints.
- Arthritis of hand joints.
- Symmetrical arthritis in at least one area.
- Rheumatoid nodules.
- Positive rheumatoid factor.
- Radiological changes.

Radiological changes that can occur with RA

- Joint erosions.
- Periarticular osteoporosis.
- Loss of joint space.
- Sublaxation.

Clinical features of RA

RA has both articular and extra-articular features as listed:
- Polyarticular swelling.
- Early morning stiffness.
- Joint pain.
- Nodules.
- Fatigue.
- Myalgia.
- Weight loss.
- Muscle wasting.
- Renal—glomerulonephritis, amyloidosis.
- Ocular—episcleritis, scleritis, Sjögren's syndrome, keratoconjunctivitis sicca.
- Cardiac—pericarditis, myocarditis, valve abnormalities.
- Pulmonary—pleural effusions, interstitial disease, nodules.
- Neurological—peripheral neuropathy.
- Vascular—vasculitis, rashes.
- Skin—rash, ulcers, vascular lesions.
- Spinal cord—cordcompression.
- Haematological—anaemia, Felty's syndrome.

Management of RA

The aim of treatment is to optimize physical, psychological, and social function and to prevent structural damage and deformity. To achieve this a multidisciplinary approach is required.

Drug therapy

The aims of drug therapy are to provide symptom relief and suppress the activity of the condition. First-line therapy consisting of analgesia and non-steroidal anti-inflammatory drugs are used to reduce pain and stiffness. Second-line therapy including, disease modifying drugs, cytotoxic and biologic therapy is used when the disease is active. It is important to commence disease modifying drugs as soon as diagnosis is confirmed to minimize structural damage and preserve function. The different disease modifying drugs include:

• Hydroxychloroquine.
• Sulfasalazine.
• Gold injections.
• Methotrexate.
• Leflunomide.
• Azathioprine.
• D-penicillamine.

Disease modifying drugs share the following characteristics
• They take 3–4 months before their efficacy can be assessed.
• All (apart from hydroxychloroquine) require regular blood tests to assess their safety.
• If monotherapy proves ineffective then combination therapy can be used.
• If the patient does not respond to two disease-modifying drugs (one of which must be methotrexate) then biologic therapy can be commenced.

For a flare of disease activity intramuscular or intravenous steroid can be administered.

Education and management

It is important that a patient learns to self manage the daily symptoms of the condition. Education can be provided in individual or group format and often involves many members of the multi-disciplinary team including

• Specialist nurse—to provide information about the condition, monitor drug therapy, provide psychological support, and advise on symptom management, e.g. fatigue and sleep disturbance. 📖 see Fibromalgia, pp.410–411 for advice regarding sleep.
• Physiotherapist—in the acute phase focus is upon reduction of pain and inflammation with hot/cold modalities (heat is useful for muscular pain and ice packs can reduce the swelling of inflamed joints), TENS (pain gating), and hydrotherapy. In the rehabilitation phase, joint protection and function are the focus with therapeutic exercise to address muscle weakness, range of movement, and pain management, assistive equipment (gait aids) and patient education. Immersion in warm wax baths can help hand pain and stiffness.
• Occupational therapist—joint protection, use of aids, splints to reduce the pain of a swollen joint, hand function, work and leisure assessment
• Podiatry—foot care, provision of orthoses and insoles to improve posture and function.

Surgery

The aim of surgery is to restore function and/or provide pain relief. Surgery is most effective when the systemic aspect of the condition is under control. The commonest surgery is hip and knee replacement. Replacement of other joints, including shoulder and elbow is also increasing. Urgent surgery is required for septic arthritis, tendon rupture, and spinal cord decompression. Due to the potential vulnerability of the cervical spine, a pre-operative spinal X-ray is required and a cervical collar may be required during surgery to remind theatre staff of the potential problems at the neck. Carpel tunnel syndrome occurs more often in patients with RA and if the symptoms are troublesome a decompression of the carpel nerve can be carried out.

Factors associated with poor prognosis include:

- High titre of rheumatoid factor.
- Many active joints at onset.
- High level of disability at onset.
- Presence of extra articular manifestations.
- Early evidence of radiological erosions.
- Low socio economic status.

Evaluating the outcome of RA

There are many tools and markers that can be used to assess the progress of RA. These include:

- The disease activity score (DAS)—this is a composite score which includes the number of swollen and tender joints, ESR, and patient global assessment using a visual analogue scale.
- Pain can be assessed using a visual analogue scale, a questionnaire such as the McGills questionnaire, or by palpating the patient's joints for tenderness—the Ritchie articular index.
- Blood markers—such as the ESR and CRP—to indicate a reduction in inflammation.
- Documenting the duration of early morning stiffness—the higher the duration the more active the condition will tend to be.
- Measuring functional ability using the Health Assessment Questionnaire which records the patient's physical ability to carry out eight aspects of daily living including dressing and personal hygiene.
- The Arthritis Impact Measurement (AIM) scales focuses on the physical, psychological, and social impact of the condition.
- The Hospital Anxiety and Depression (HAD) scale assess the psychological impact of the condition.

Inflammatory arthritis— spondyloarthropathies

Definition

The spondyloarthropathies are a group of inflammatory arthritides affecting the spine, sacroiliac joints, peripheral joints and entheses. Conditions involved in this group are shown in Table 26.1.

Causes

- Human leucocyte antigen B27 is a genetic risk factor.
- Different types of spondyloarthropathies can be found in members of the same family.
- In reactive arthritis infection is the major cause with the condition triggered by gastroenteritis or urethritis.

Investigations

- Haematology—indicators of inflammation and acute phase response e.g. ESR, full blood count.
- Immunology—HLA B27; autoantibodies to rule out other diagnoses.
- Biochemistry—liver, bone, urea and electrolytes, CRP.
- Microbiology—urethral swabs.
- Joint aspiration.
- Radiological investigations.

Clinical features

See Table 26.2

Treatments for spondyloarthropathies

- *Drug therapy*—to relieve symptoms, analgesia, non-steroidal anti-inflammatory drugs, antibiotics for reactive arthritis, intra-muscular or intra-articular corticosteroid injections. To suppress disease activity-disease modifying drugs and biologic agents.
- *Physiotherapy*—all patients require daily exercises to maintain function, posture and spinal movement. Ideally this should be done with the support of a physiotherapist. Hydrotherapy is a good medium to improve muscle strength and range of movement. Ultrasound can help with enthesitis and TENs assists some patients in pain management.
- *Surgery*—the most common intervention is hip arthroplasty especially for AS patients. Knee and shoulder replacements can also be required.

Table 26.1 Spondyloarthropathic prevalence and sex ratio in the UK

	Prevalence in UK	Sex ratio (male: female)
Ankylosing spondylitis (AS)	150 per 100 000	4:1
Psoriatic arthritis	100 per 100 000	1:1
Reactive arthritis	30 per 100 000	3:1
Enteropathic arthritis	–	1:1

Table 26.2 Clinical features of spondyloarthropathies

Spondyloarthropathy	Features
Ankylosing spondylitis	Low back and buttock pain
	Peripheral arthritis
	Iritis
	Enthesis
	Reduced chest expansion
Reactive arthritis	Urethritis/gastroenteritis
	Lower limb arthritis
	Triad of arthritis, conjunctivitis and urethritis
	Enthesis
	Inflammatory spinal pain
	Keratoderma blenorrhagica
	Amyloidosis
Psoriatic arthritis	Psorasis
	Monoarthritis or dactylitis ('sausage toe')
	Inflammatory spinal pain
	Enthesis
	Nail changes
	Amylodosis
	Arthritis in several joints
Enteropathic arthritis	Bowel disease
	Lower limb peripheral arthritis
	Spinal pain
	Enthesis
	Tendonitis

Chronic pain conditions—osteoarthritis

Osteoarthritis (OA) is the most common condition to affect the synovial joints and is the main cause of locomotor disability.

Definition

OA use to be considered a degenerative condition but our present understanding is that a metabolic process is occurring, affecting the synovial joints, with focal cartilage loss and a reparative bone response.

Risk factors for OA include:

- Age—OA is uncommon in those <45 years.
- Sex—females more likely to experience hand and knee OA.
- Occupation—farmers associated with hip OA.
- Genetic—inherited component to hand, knee and hip OA.
- Lifestyle—e.g. obesity.

Diagnosis

- The diagnosis of OA is based on clinical and radiological findings—laboratory tests are normal.
- Plain X-rays show joint space narrowing, osteophytes, subchondral cysts, and bone cysts.
- Often too much importance is given to radiographic change and a poor correlation exists between structural changes and symptoms.
- Analysis of synovial fluid can also be useful.

Clinical features of OA

OA commonly affects the hips, knees, distal interphalangeal joints (DIPs), thumb joint (first carpometacarpal joint), lower cervical spine and first metatarsophalangeal joint. Clinical features the patient may experience include:

- Pain on activity.
- Post activity stiffness.
- Joint swelling.
- Reduced joint function.
- Bony enlargement.
- Joint instability.
- Joint effusion.
- Gait abnormalities.
- Heberden's nodes on DIPs.
- Bouchard's nodes.
- Crepitus.
- Restricted joint movement.
- Muscle weakness and wasting.

Secondary causes of OA

- Metabolic/endocrine—haemachromatosis, acromegly, hyperparathyroidism.
- Neuropathic disorder—diabetes mellitus.
- Inflammatory arthritis—RA, gout, septic arthritis.
- Anatomical abnormalities—bone dysplasia.

- Developmental—hypermobility, congenital dislocation of the hip, perthes disease, epiphyseal dysplasias.
- Mechanical—obesity, trauma, previous joint surgery.

Management of OA

The aims of treatment include: educating the patient so self management strategies can be adopted; pain management; and maintaining function. The misconception that OA is due to ageing often leads to patients believing that little can be done when in fact, their are many coping strategies that the patient can engage in. A patient's mood is an important factor in determining how successfully symptoms are managed and should be assessed along with sleep during the assessment process and treatment advocated if necessary (☐ see p.412). Consequently it is important to involve the patient in all aspects of care management so that they can become an active participant in their care.

Drug management

Paracetamol is the drug of choice and the patient may need educating on the benefits of taking paracetamol at regular intervals to achieve maximum effect. Topical non-steroidal drugs or capsaicin can be useful for hand and knee OA. If oral non-steroidal drugs are required they should be used for a short time span and at a low dose during a flare of the symptoms. Non-steroidal drugs are not recommended for use in elderly patients. Some studies have demonstrated improvement with the use of the health supplement glucosamine in knee OA only. Joint aspiration and injection with corticosteroid can be used for knee effusions.

Exercise

The most helpful advice to give a patient with OA is to carry out regular exercise. Many patients are fearful that exercise will increase their pain and lead to the affected joint 'wearing out'. It is important to reassure the patient that this is not the case and in fact a reduction in activity will lead to an escalation of their symptoms. The type of exercise that is required includes strengthening exercises for specific joints as well as advice on aerobic exercise to improve stamina and fatigue. Exercise can also help with weight reduction, joint proprioception, and psychological status. The Arthritis and Research Campaign produce a range of educational booklets that provide advice on exercise.[1]

Reducing of biomechanical stress

- Weight reduction can reduce pain and improve stamina and general levels of fitness.
- Insoles and the use of shoes with deep cushioning—such as trainers—can redistribute stress and reduce impact loading.
- The use of walking sticks and other mobility aids need to be considered to improve function.
- Increased muscle balance (length/strength) around affected joints will support biomechanical alignment.

Surgery

- Surgery should be considered for patients with uncontrolled pain, especially at night and limitation in function.
- Hip and knee replacements can greatly improve a person's quality of life.
- Surgery has also become more common on shoulder, elbow and thumb joints.

References

1. www.arc.org.uk

Chronic pain conditions—fibromyalgia

Definition

A condition characterized by widespread musculoskeletal pain, non restorative sleep, fatigue, and a host of other physical and psychological associations.

Incidence

Fibromyalgia occurs in 0.5% of men and 3.4% of women. The onset in women usually occurs between 25–45 years. Fibromyalgia is the third commonest reason to be referred to a rheumatologist.

Cause

No single pathophysiological causative mechanism has been identified and it would appear that fibromyalgia is a multifactorial syndrome. Fibromyalgia can be associated with other musculoskeletal conditions such as rheumatoid arthritis where it is referred to as 'secondary fibromyalgia'.
Possible causes of fibromyalgia include:
- Abnormal pain processing.
- Sleep disturbance.
- Muscle pathology.
- Genetic predisposition to pain sensitivity.
- Neurohormonal dysfunction.
- Neuroendocrine disturbances.
- Neurotransmitter regulation.
- Allergy, infection, toxicity, and nutritional deficiency.
- Physical trauma-RTA, whiplash.
- Emotional trauma.

Diagnosis

In 1990 the American College of Rheumatology developed criteria for fibromyalgia for research purposes (Box 26.3). In clinical practice the diagnosis is made on the basis of the clinical history and examination.

Clinical features from the history

- Widespread musculoskeletal pain.
- Pain is a constant feature.
- Tired all the time.
- Joint stiffness.
- Non restorative sleep.
- Difficulty carrying out normal activities.

Other physical and psychological associations include:

- Physical associations:
  - Irritable bowel.
  - Irritable bladder.
  - Temperature changes.
  - Paraesthesia.
  - Perception of swelling.
  - Migraine.
  - Muscle spasm.
  - Dizziness.

- Psychological associations
  - Panic attacks
  - Anxiety
  - Depression
  - Irritability
  - Memory lapses
  - Word mix ups
  - Reduced concentration.

Box 26.3 The American College of Rheumatology criteria for fibromyalgia

- Widespread musculoskeletal pain in all four quadrants of the body and some axial pain (cervical spine, anterior chest, thoracic spine or low back).
- Pain present for at least 3 months.
- Hyperlagesic points on digital pressure of 4 kgs in 11 out of 18 sites on the body.

The points are all bilateral and situated in:
- Suboccipital muscle insertions at the base of the skull.
- Low cervical spine C5–C7 interspinous ligaments.
- Trapezius muscles at the midpoint of the upper boarder.
- Supraspinatus origins above the scapulae spines.
- Second costochondral junctions on upper surface lateral to junction 2 cm distal to lateral epicondyles.
- Upper outer quadrant of buttock in anterior folds of gluteus medius.
- Greater trochanters posterior to trochanteric prominence.
- Medial fat pads of knee proximal to the joint line.

Examination

The main finding is the presence of symmetrical tender/painful sites around the body. In patients without fibromyalgia these sites are uncomfortable to firm pressure but in patients with fibromyalgia the same pressure causes the patient to cry out and withdraw the area being examined.

Investigations

Limited investigations are required to exclude other causes for the symptoms. Polymyalgia rheumatica, spondylarthropathy and hypothyroidism can also give rise to similar symptoms. Investigations include:
- Full blood count.
- Inflammatory markers e.g. ESR and CRP.
- Biochemical profile-serum calcium, alkaline phosphatase, creatine kinase, blood sugar.
- Thyroid function tests.

It is important to make a diagnosis of fibromyalgia after the clinical history and examination and explain to the patient that the blood tests are simply to ensure there is no underlying condition. Radiological investigations are not required.

Chronic pain conditions—management

There are similarities between patients with fibromyalgia, repetitive strain injury, chronic back pain, chronic fatigue syndrome, and reflex sympathetic dystrophy (RSD). Therefore a common approach to management can be applied. The main goals of management include:
- To optimize physical, psychological, and social function.
- To help patient develop self management/coping skills.

The Arthritis and Musculoskeletal Alliance (ARMA), British Society of Rheumatology, and the Pain Society have all produced evidence-based guidelines which can be accessed online.[1–3]

Education

The patient will need guidance, support and motivation from a health professional before feeling able to take an active role in the management of their symptoms. Useful patient websites are listed in the reference section.[4–6]

Patient-centred management goals need to be realistic, achievable, and meaningful for the patient to engage in. Patients who utilize active rather than passive coping strategies report less pain-related disability and distress, better general health, and use fewer health care services and medications.

Active strategies are those that involve some action by the individual to manage their pain through their own efforts whereas passive strategies refer to an individual who is more reliant on the efforts of others or depend on medications.

The current evidence advocates the use of behavioural strategies including:
- Graded exercise.
- Pacing.
- Cognitive behavioural therapy (CBT).
- Goal setting.
- Relaxation.
- Stress management.

Some of these strategies are covered in chronic disease management programmes such as the Expert Patient Programmes.

There is no evidence that one specific behavioural approach is more effective than another but treatment is likely to be more effective if it:
- Includes more than education alone.
- Includes teaching patients skills based on rehearsal or practice.
- Is aimed at changing behaviour and improving function.

CBT
- This is a widely used form of psychotherapy which aims to identify and change maladaptive patterns of thought and behaviour.
- CBT can help patients adjust to their illness and acquire skills that can be used in their daily routine and is most effective for patients who experience significant problems with daily emotional, household, social, or work related function.

- CBT can improve a patient's sense of control regarding their symptoms. Aspects such as relapse prevention should be included in the CBT programme.
- CBT for persistent pain should be applied early in the development of problems with daily functioning and not as a last resort.
- More intensive courses of CBT are more effective. The choice between less intensive, unidisciplinary outpatient-based courses versus intense multidisciplinary residential or hospital-based courses should be made on the basis of the impact of the condition. If a patient has been out of work for an extended period, lost the structure of the day, and if their mood and symptoms predominate and dictate their activities an intense course of multidisciplinary input would be beneficial.

Improving sleep

Patients often experience a disturbed sleep pattern and feel unrefreshed on waking. This increases the perception of pain, leading to low mood, reduced cognitive functioning, and a reduced ability to manage the symptoms. Self help measures should be advocated including:

- Developing a sleep routine—going to bed at the same time each night and avoiding day time sleeping.
- Avoiding stimulants such as coffee.
- Carrying out relaxation techniques to clear the mind.
- Ensuring that the bedroom is quiet and well ventilated.

Tricyclics can be useful in helping improve sleep. Numbers needed to treat are n=4. The most commonly prescribed tricyclic is amitriptyline. This is prescribed in small incremental doses ranging from 10–50mgs and should be taken 2–4 hours before settling. The decision regarding dosage will be based on efficacy and side effects. Tricyclics should help to improve sleep within 2–3 weeks but take 3–4 months before modifying pain perception.

Exercise

Many patients become less physically active due to the pain and are fearful that movement will increase the symptoms of pain and fatigue. Graded exercise is advocated to recondition the body and to improve muscle stamina, strength, stiffness, and generalized fitness. Graded exercise involves gradually increasing activity over a period of time. Several sessions of supervised exercise by the physiotherapy may be needed to provide motivation, education, reassurance, and feedback.

Relaxation

- Patient can be taught relaxation techniques to help with:
- Muscle tension
- Anxiety
- Sleep
- Foster a sense of control over symptoms

Pacing

Pacing involves breaking down everyday activities into achievable components. Patients tend to exert themselves on a 'good day' and under exert on a 'poor day'. If patients can plan their activities—e.g. cleaning one room in the house a day instead of doing all the rooms in one go—they will still achieve their goal and be active every day. Patients should always be encouraged to remain in the workplace and where possible apply the principles of pacing in the work situation.

Managing depression

Symptoms of depression are common in chronic musculoskeletal pain conditions.
- For mild depression CBT, exercise, relaxation and pacing techniques can all be considered.
- For moderate-to-severe depression the selective serotonin reuptake inhibitors (SSRIs) should be the first option.
  - Citalopram 20mg daily is often considered the drug of choice as it is well tolerated, has few side effects and few drug interactions. Patients should be told that it will take 2 weeks before the drug becomes effective.
  - Antidepressants also have analgesic effects which can be very useful when treating this group of patients although no antidepressant is currently licensed for the management of chronic musculoskeletal pain in the UK.
  - If a patient does not respond to antidepressant treatment then a psychiatric referral should be considered.

Other pharmacological options for the management of chronic musculoskeletal pain

- Paracetamol.
- If paracetamol is not effective add in codeine phosphate.
- If codeine is not tolerated or ineffective meptazinol, nefopam, or tramadol may be considered but there is little evidence to support the use of strong narcotics. There are concerns with tramadol as it can cause patients to become dependant on it and therefore should be used with caution in patients who have a history of dependence or addiction. It can also interact with the SSRIs and the tricyclics to cause convulsions.
- Duloxetine has been shown to reduce pain in women with fibromyalgia.
- Pregabalin has been shown to reduce pain, fatigue and improve sleep.

Complementary/alterative medicine (CAM)

While few studies have examined the benefits of CAM, patients often use numerous types of complementary/alternative medicine including massage therapy, chiropractic treatment and acupuncture.

References

1. ⁻ᵈ www.arma.uk.net
2. ⁻ᵈ www.britishpainsociety.org
3. ⁻ᵈ www.rheumatology.org.uk
4. ⁻ᵈ www.dipex.org/EXEC
5. ⁻ᵈ www.britishpainsociety.org/patient_home.htm
6. ⁻ᵈ www.expertpatients.nhs.uk
7. ⁻ᵈ www.arc.org.uk

Further reading

1. Hakin A, Clunie G, and Hakim A (2006). *The Oxford Handbook of Rheumatology*, 2ⁿᵈ edn. Oxford University Press, Oxford.
2. Snaith M (2004). *ABC of Rheumatology*, 3ʳᵈ edn. BMJ Books, London.
3. Main C and Spanswick C (2000). *Pain Management: An interdisciplinary approach*. Churchill Livingstone, Edinburgh.

Spinal pain and soft tissue rheumatism

Introduction

Low back and neck pain are common and may result from abnormalities occurring within the vertebrae, the intervertebral discs, the facet joints, the ligaments and from the spinal canal and the nerve roots themselves. Pain may be referred from distant sites—such as the abdomen—and in some cases may be functional or psychogenic in nature.

Acute back pain

Causes

- Muscular or ligamentous strain.
- Intervertebral disc prolapse.
- Facet joint dysfunction.
- Bony trauma.
- Acute inflammatory disease or infection (joint or bony).
- Tumours.

Acute pain de novo usually presents to rheumatologists or orthopaedic surgeons rather then to a physician in Rehabilitation Medicine in the UK and this topic is better addressed in rheumatological and orthopaedic texts. The treatment of back pain has been described in the Clinical Standards Advisory Group (CSAG) guidelines[1] and bedrest is nowadays not recommended for acute simple low back pain. Short-term rest may be useful for some patients in the case of intervertebral disc prolapse, when pain may be referred to the leg by nerve root entrapment. When this occurs in a true spinal root distribution it is known as sciatica, but the term should not be applied to other referred pain in the leg and back.

It is important to identify the patient's description of pain. He or she may often describe symptoms as hip pain while pointing to the buttock and it is important to distinguish one from the other. Pain from the hip is usually in the groin or near the trochanter whereas spinal pain is found in the buttock or trochanter. Patients may be quite vague about the distribution of any leg pain and it is important to try to pin the patient down to specific symptoms. Knowledge of the spine's anatomy and of the typical radiation patterns of pain are therefore important.

Management

Acute pain usually resolves spontaneously after a few days or weeks, but, if it persists, further investigation should be carried out to exclude an underlying inflammatory lesion or neoplasia. Treatment should go along the following lines:

- Analgesics.
- Imaging in simple acute back pain is usually unhelpful, but may give an indication of previous underlying disease, such as lumbar spondylosis or osteoporosis.
- Leg pain and sciatica may be helped by a lumbar or caudal epidural injection.
- Acute exacerbation of facet joint pain, in which there is a local tenderness of one and no more than two joints, eased by local infiltration of corticosteroid and local anaesthetic.
- Mobilizing exercises have been shown to be useful and no specific technique has been shown to better than any other. The aim is to relieve the pressure on the spinal structures and rest and cessation of the incriminating factors will usually settle the situation.
- Use of isokinetic devices to help restore mechanical function appears to be useful, but needs further study.

References

1. Clinical Standards Advisory Group (1994). *CSAG Report on Back Pain*. HMSO, London.

Chronic back pain

Causes
- Posture.
- Facet joint pain.
- Short leg syndrome.
- Lumbar spondylosis.
- Degenerative disc disease.
- Spondylolisthesis and spondylolysis.
- Diffuse idiopathic skeletal hyperostosis.
- Spinal stenosis.

Posture
Prolonged poor posture alters the normal curve of the spine and stresses the structures therein.

Short leg syndrome
Unequal leg lengths tilt the pelvis, produce a scoliosis in the spine and strain ligaments and joints. Correcting the leg length difference may be helpful.

Prolapsed intervertebral disc (Table 27.1) Facet joint pain
Well-defined back pain syndrome associated with lumbar spondylosis. Pain is experienced on extension of the spine, both in an upright position and in sitting, and can be provoked on bending forwards. The pain often radiates to the buttock or into the sacrum and may extend down the leg but rarely extends beyond the knee. This is not nerve root pain.

Spondylosis
Dysfunction of vertebral structures causes a chronic low grade pain. This is the end result of degenerative changes in the spine and occurs at points of movement of the spine (facet joints and vertebral bodies).

Spondylolisthesis and spondylolysis
This is a displacement of one vertebra on another—usually an anterior movement of a vertebra above on the one below, but posterior movement of the vertebra above on that below can also occur and is referred to as retrolisthesis. Spondylolysis occurs when the spondylolisthesis is caused by a defect in the pars interarticularis in the vertebral lamina. The symptoms are very similar to that of facet joint pain.

Spinal stenosis
Chronic narrowing of the spinal spinal canal or foramen, which usually occurs as a result of chronic degenerative disease following recurrent disc prolapse and loss of disc height or by facet joint arthritis impinging into the spinal canal. Back and leg pain occur with physical activity and then settle at rest in most patients. It is also found that flexion of the spine relieves the symptoms and walking up hills and going up stairs is often more comfortable than on the flat or going downhill. MRI is diagnostic at confirming the level of narrowing and a laminectomy is the treatment of choice.

Table 27.1 Prolapsed intervertebral disc and effects

Disc prolapse	Affectd nerve root	Loss of reflex	Dermatome	Typical muscle weakness
L3/4	L4	Knee jerk	Anterior aspect of knee and medial aspect of lower leg down to ankle.	Quadriceps, part of tibialis anterior, tibialis posterior
L4/5	L5		Postero-lateral aspect of thigh, lateral aspect of lower leg, dorsum and medial aspect of foot including the medial 3½ toes.	Foot dorsiflexors and evertors. Tibialis posterior
L5/S1	S1	Ankle jerk	Small strip of posterior aspect of thigh and posterior aspect of calf, heel and lateral aspect of foot including lateral 1½ toes.	Foot plantar flexors, lateral hamstrings and thigh abductors (gluteus maximus)

Specific management (Table 27.2)

Table 27.2 Specific management of chronic back pain

Condition	Treatment
Posture	Analgesics; treat the underlying cause.
Short leg syndrome	Correct the leg length difference with either an insole or shoe raise.
Prolapsed disc	Most settle spontaneously with rest, but the biomechanical effect on the facet joints must be addressed. Discectomy for intractible nerve root compression.
Facet joint pain	Analgesia; joint injection.
Spondylosis	Analgesia for acute pain, hydrotherapy for stiffness. (📖 see p.160)
Spondylolisthesis/lysis	Treatment usually conservative. Immobilization of the spine for bad symptoms or for nerve root compression. Spinal fusion may be a definitive procedure.
Spinal stenosis	Laminectomy ± foraminal decompression is the treatment of choice.

Pain management

Patient education and the development of a realistic approach to lifestyle management are important. Treat acute painful exacerbations. Suitable regimen of analgesics and therapies is required for background pain. Direct management to social and occupational needs rather than search for a cure (☐ discussed in Chapter 13, p.183). The patient should be taught mild, gentle, but effective exercise by a physiotherapist to improve muscle strength and to mobilize the spine. Thereafter, the patient should be expected to continue the exercises—particularly during quiescent periods. Warm water exercises in a local swimming pool are valuable in providing heat and a medium in which exercise can be done.

Lifestyle management is the rewarding aspect of rehabilitation. Psychological advice may identify the key issues producing the symptoms in some patients with clear instructions on how to manage daily routines and deal with acute exacerbations. Patients and relatives must be given consistent messages for successful outcomes. Therapy should be reserved for acute exacerbations, for which there should be clear indications. The specialist team should also involve the primary care team, Social Services, and the Disability Employment Adviser. Alterations to the home, workplace, and transportation are important and back pain sufferers should be encouraged to take up activities, which will not cause particularly difficulties for their symptoms.

Neck pain

- Neck pain is common and the principles of management are similar to that of managing back pain (📖 see Acute back pain, p. 420; Chronic back pain, p. 422).
- Acute exacerbations are a common feature of chronic neck pain. Symptom duration following injury depends on severity but should settle within a few weeks in the absence of disruption of the ligamentous structures to the spine.
- Neck pain of mechanical origin usually produces asymmetric restriction of movement, whereas neck pain of inflammatory origin (e.g. rheumatoid disease, ankylosing spondylitis) tends to be symmetrical.

Clinical features

- Acute exacerbations—most last for no more than a few days and are often associated with some unaccustomed activity, awkward posture/injury.
- Pain and stiffness—back of lower neck; radiates to occiput, down spine, shoulders/down arms. Usually aggravated by movement of the neck and relieved by rest.
- Nerve root compression—may occur, most commonly in C7 dermatome.
- Whiplash injury—anterior neck pain may be present for several months. The absence of nerve root involvement and a full range of neck movements on active and passive examination would suggest complete resolution of the neck pain symptoms. These would not be expected to persist for >2 years or give rise to subsequent degenerative change.
- See Table 27.3 for symptoms and signs and Table 27.4 for distribution of neck pain.

Symptoms in mechanical causes

- Intermittent.
- Pain confined to articular and dural distribution.
- Neurological features confined to a single root.

Red flags

- Constant or progressive symptoms.
- Bilateral neurological signs or involving > one nerve root.

Table 27.3 Symptoms and signs of neck pain

Problem	Symptoms	Signs
Articular	Intermittent neck pain	Asymmetrical restriction of neck movement
Dural	Occiput, vertex, scapula, shoulder and interscapular pain	Pain may occur on shoulder adduction or external rotation, but pain on forced lateral flexion of cervical spine
Nerve Root	Severe pain in appropriate dermatome	Weakness and sensory impairment in affected nerve root distribution, abnormal reflex if necessary

Table 27.4 Neck distribution of neck pain

Root	Pain distribution	Muscle weakness	Tendon Reflex
C2	Occiput radiating over head to forehead Neck, jaw, and cheek		
C3			
C4	Trapezius and upper medial border of scapula		
C5	Shoulder tip, lateral side of upper arm	Supraspinatus, infraspinatus, deltoid, biceps	Biceps
C6	Front of arm, lateral aspect of elbow, and radial border of forearm down to thumb	Biceps, supinator	Supinator
C7	Middle of anterior and posterior aspects of forearm, middle and ring fingers	Triceps, wrist flexors	Triceps
C8	Ulnar aspect of forearm and hand, ring, and little finger	Wrist and finger flexors, thumb flexors	
T1	Medial aspect of elbow. Upper pectoral and mid scapula areas	Intrinsic hand muscles	
T2	Medial aspect of upper arm and axilla		

Treatment

Analgesics and rest—perhaps with use of a soft collar to maintain a neutral position—can be helpful. There is considerable debate about whether collars are helpful or harmful. There is no doubt that they have a place in providing some short-term relief for patients with acute exacerbations of chronic neck pain and their main benefit comes from intermittent use, even in some cases nocturnal usage. Collars also have their place for short-term use after acute injuries, but in the long term they can produce stiffness and lost movement in the spine, which can allow the patient to develop unnecessary longer lasting symptoms. If there is a risk of neurological injury, then a collar is mandatory to restrict movements. They are also of importance in patients with severe erosive rheumatoid disease going for surgery, even if they do not have gross cervical spine disease. This alerts the anaesthetist to the risk of cord damage from neck extension during intubation. The aim is to restrict neck movements to about one third, and, while rigid collars can achieve reduction to about 10%, they are cumbersome and uncomfortable to wear. They should thus be reserved for patients at risk of neurological compression.

Physical

Physiotherapy and chiropracty are commonly performed. Traction can be used when root pain occurs in either a lying or sitting position. There is evidence to support the use of manual techniques over exercise in decreasing pain and maintaining range of movement. Mobilization exercises and manipulation are also performed where cervical joints are repeatedly pressed through their ranges of movement. Manipulation is simply a more energetic and aggressive form of mobilization, but older patients should not generally be subjected to it. Patients with chronic pain may also respond to both TENS and acupuncture, which have a useful carry over effect after its use.

Medication

Analgesics and anti-inflammatories are the mainstay of treatment in acute neck pain. There is no good evidence for the effectiveness of the latter in mechanical and degenerative disease, but the reality is that patients feel that they are helpful. For the most part, patients are usually managed with a combination of analgesics and physical treatments, but in some cases this is not enough. Mood changes quite quickly on the realisation that the pain has started to persist and the addition of a tricyclic antidepressant is helpful. The evidence points to the latter being more effective than other types, although in reality, both these and selective serotonin uptake inhibitors have wide usage. Gabapentin and pregabalin are also increasingly used for a wide variety of pain and there is good evidence for its effect on neurogenic pain. Topical medication is not helpful in neck pain, as creams do not have enough penetration to reach even down to the underlying muscles.

Surgery

In degenerative disease, surgery is primarily indicated to decompress the spinal cord or nerve roots or to fuse the spine for instability. An anterior approach (Cloward's procedure) is favoured over a posterior. The results of surgery are good in well-selected patients and most resume their previous lifestyles.

Because neck pain can become chronic and very disabling, many other associated features can develop, which are discussed further in 📖 Chapter 11, p.160.

Further reading

1. Braddom RL (2006). *Physical Medicine and Rehabilitation*, 3rd edn. WB Saunders, Philadelphia.

Shoulder pain

The upper limb is suspended from the trunk by muscular attachments and thus any condition affecting muscular strength or function may cause pain affecting the shoulder (gleno-humeral) joint itself, the acromio-clavicular joint, or the rotator cuff group of muscles. In addition, degenerative disease in the neck, brachial plexus dysfunction, trapezius muscle spasm, diaphragmatic and pericardial conditions may cause referred shoulder pain, but these will not be considered in detail here. The skin around the shoulder is supplied by the C5 root, which will lead to shoulder muscle (rotator cuff) weakness when damaged, as well as sensory disturbance over the point of the shoulder.

Pain may occur either as a result of inflammation, impingement of the rotator cuff tendons, or as a result of a tendon tear. Impingement occurs when the sliding movement of the supraspinatus tendon is restricted as it passes under the acromio clavicular joint or coracoid-acromial ligament. Shoulder pain classically occurs on movement or when lying on the affected side at night. The 'painful arc syndrome' causes discomfort as the shoulder is raised in abduction and, as the movement continues, the pain then disappears. Pain in the impingement syndrome is usually brought on internal rotation and flexion of the upper arm and can be elicited by asking the patient to place the hand on the opposite shoulder and to push the elbow forward. A rotator cuff tendon tear usually results in pain and weakness of the relevant tendon's movement.

A shoulder must keep moving to maintain function and a fall may produce supraspinatus tendon damage and extreme pain, such that the patient stops moving the limb. The restriction of movement can lead very quickly on to a true frozen shoulder, i.e. an adhesive capsulitis. Three distinct syndromes exist in the painful shoulder:

Rotator cuff lesions

May occur in degenerative change or following an injury, e.g. falling onto an outstretched hand (◻ see Table 27.5). A rotator cuff syndrome may occur as a result of vascular changes and mechanical factors affecting normal muscular and tendon function which produces pain. Over time, the space between the acromion process and the glenohumeral joint diminishes leading particularly to restriction of the supraspinatus tendon and an impingement syndrome. The various elements of the rotator cuff syndrome are discussed next:

Supraspinatus tendinitis

Affects the supraspinatus mechanism closest to its insertion into the greater tuberosity and pain and limitation of active and passive abduction are characteristic. A painful arc occurs on abduction between 90° and 120°. The pain may be increased on resisting abduction of the arm in the first 15° of movement by placing the examiner's hand on the elbow and asking the patient to abduct the arm against the examiner's hand on the elbow. Some cases occur acutely and are associated with calcium deposits, (seen on X-ray). Injection into the subacromial bursa is the medical treatment of choice.

Infraspinatus/subscapularis tendinitis

Although less common than supraspinatus tendinitis, these two lesions give distinctive features. Both cause pain on abduction of the arm, but the former gives rise to pain on external rotation of the arm and the latter to pain on internal rotation of the arm. The former is more common in sportsmen than other lesions of the rotator cuff.

Bicipital tendinitis

This produces pain anteriorly on the shoulder in the area where the bicipital tendon passes through the groove in the humeral head to attach in the coracoid process. Local injection is helpful.

Subacromial bursitis

This somewhat non-specific term describes a rotator cuff problem, where the specific tendon lesion is not readily identifiable. The pain is evident on shoulder abduction and flexion and both may be restricted. Stressing the individual tendons may not produce intense pain in one area more than in others. The most common feature is a painful arc around 60–120° of abduction.

Table 27.5 Rotator cuff muscles

Muscle	Action	Innervation
Deltoid	Abduction and flexion of arm 15–90°	Axillary N.
Supraspinatus	Abduction of arm 0–15° and 90° upwards	Suprascapular N.
Infraspinatus	External rotation of arm	Suprascapular N.
Subscapularis	Internal rotation of arm	Suprascapular N.
Serratus anterior	Protraction of arm	Long thoracic N.
Biceps brachii long head	Forearm supination, elbow/shoulder flexion	Musculocutaneous N.
Pectoralis major	Adduction of arm	Long thoracic N.
Teres major and minor	Adduction of arm	Axillary N.
Latissimus dorsi	Adduction of arm from 60°	
Rhomboids	Shoulder extension	

N, nerve.

Adhesive capsulitis—frozen shoulder

Occurs following trauma, following rotator cuff lesions, or immobility from other causes, e.g. stroke, chest surgery, and pathology (myocardial infarction, pericarditis, and particularly sternal splits). It may be spontaneous and is more common in diabetics. The essential feature is an inflamed gleno-humeral capsule, which eventually shrinks and thickens, thus restricting movement. Abduction is restricted in common with rotator cuff lesions, but the pathognomonic feature is loss of external rotation. Early treatment is important, as a secondary reflex sympathetic dystrophy can occur, leading to a useless arm and hand, which will be very difficult to treat.

Acromioclavicular joint lesions

Develops in people in their 40s and 50s due to joint degeneration. There is joint tenderness and pain on stressing flexion and abduction of the arm between 60–90°. Radiographs show loss of joint space and possibly osteo-phytes, which may cause an impingement syndrome by inferior projection.

Treatment of shoulder pain

Treatment of these lesions is essentially with analgesics and physiotherapy to mobilize the joint. NSAIDs are of little use and it may be necessary to use quite strong analgesics to allow sleep. Rotator cuff lesions may respond to an injection of steroid and local anaesthetic into the subacromial bursa and adhesive capsulitis responds by the similar infiltration into the gleno-humeral joint itself. If rotator cuff lesions persist and are clearly due to impingement, it may be necessary after MR scanning to decompress the space surgically. Injection of the acromioclavicular joint can be very effective if the pain emanates from there. Similarly, the distal end of the clavicle may require removal in persistent severe acromioclavicular joint pain.

The principle of treating adhesive capsulitis is to mobilize the joint physically and to utilize injections to allow physical treatment to be taken further. If this is not possible, manipulation of the joint under anaesthetic has no proven effect, but is useful in some patients, as long as an intensive series of physiotherapy treatments is planned for 5 days immediately after the procedure. The prognosis is in fact very good for all these lesions.

Surgery is the treatment of choice for rotator cuff impingement through division of the coracoid-acromial ligament or, in more severe cases, through removal of the lower half of the acromioclavicular joint with its osteophytes. Full thickness tendon tears require repair, but most partial tears will probably repair spontaneously. Corticosteroid injections may interfere with the healing process and should be avoided in most cases. Gentle strengthening of the other rotator cuff muscles will protect the damaged tendon and accelerate healing.

Lateral humeral epicondylitis (tennis elbow) and medial humeral epicondylitis (golfer's elbow)

Two annoying conditions in people over the age of 40—thought to be part of an upper limb overuse syndrome resulting from excessive tension on the common forearm extensor and flexor muscles respectively, which results in localized tenderness and pain on gripping and twisting the hand (Box 27.1). They often prevent function of the hand, particularly in lifting weights. May be associated with neck pain.

> ### Box 27.1 Definitions
>
> *Tennis elbow*
> - Tender lateral humeral epicondyle.
> - Epicondylar pain on resisting wrist or finger extension supporting arm (straight elbow).
> - Forced pronation of the forearm with the elbow straight also produces pain.
>
> *Golfer's elbow*
> - Tender medial humeral epicondyle.
> - Epicondylar pain on resisting wrist or finger flexion supporting arm (straight elbow).
> - Pain on resisted supination less reliable.
> - Sensory symptoms do not typically occur.

Atypical epicondylitis features
- Bilateral symptoms and signs, or the presence of both golfer's and tennis elbow.
- No epicondylar tenderness.
- Paraesthesiae in the arm and painful limitation of neck movements, associated with nerve root disturbance.
- Failure to respond to local injection or occurrence within a week or two of injection.
- Clinical or radiological evidence of arthritis at the elbow.

Treatment
Physical treatment is usually helpful in mild cases. No one particular treatment has been shown to be superior to another. An epicondylitis clasp worn reasonably tightly around the upper forearm just below the common extensor or common flexor origin can protect the common muscular origin by transmitting forces away from the enthesis (where the tendon attaches to bone). This can usefully allow people to continue to work. If these measures are not sufficient, local injection of hydrocortisone is very useful in diminishing and treating symptoms. Hydrocortisone alone should be used in preference to fluorinated corticosteroids, as the latter may cause subcutaneous fat atrophy and local disfigurement.

Carpal tunnel syndrome

This is due to entrapment of the median nerve as it passes through the carpal tunnel under the flexor retinaculum at the wrist (Box 27.2). It is usually idiopathic and may be associated with expansion of the long flexor tendons, but may occur secondarily to other conditions.

> **Box 27.2 Causes**
> - Fluid retention—pregnancy or oral contraceptive—commonest association.
> - Osteoarthritis or rheumatoid arthritis of the wrist.
> - Colles and scaphoid bone fractures.
> - Direct trauma.
> - Hypothyroidism.
> - Acromegaly.
> - Amyloidosis.
> - Scheie's syndrome.
> - Myelomatosis.

Mild carpal tunnel syndrome

Features

Pain and paraesthesiae occurring in the territory of the median nerve (i.e. radial aspect of the palmar surface of the hand to include the lateral 3½ fingers). Nocturnal pain and causing patients to wake and gain relief by hanging their hand out of bed (cools the limb and reduces symptoms).

Treatment

Resting wrist in a volar splint to prevent excessive extension and flexion. Local hydrocortisone injectionsindicated if splinting alone insufficient.

More severe carpal tunnel syndrome

Features

Motor involvement occurs with abductor pollicis brevis weakness and atrophy.

Treatment

Decompression of the carpal tunnel (particularly where active denervation is present) by removal of a strip of the flexor retinaculum. Good prognosis.

The diagnosis is made by examination and confirmed by a positive *Tinel's sign* where percussion of the nerve at the wrist produces pain and paraesthesiae in the median nerve territory. A similar result may also be achieved by sustained full flexion or extension of the wrist (*Phalen's sign*). Nerve conduction studies and electromyography of the abductor pollicis brevis muscle give the diagnosis and locates the site of the median nerve compression.

De Quervain's stenosing tenosynovitis

Pain and tenderness on the radial aspect of the wrist due to inflammation of abductor pollicis longus and extensor pollicis brevis tendon sheaths. Occupational activity is often responsible and a positive Finkelstein's test is indicative. This is carried out by flexion and opposition of the thumb into the palm of the hand and held down by the fingers. The wrist is then subjected to an ulnar deviation force, thus stretching the affected tendons and producing pain. Treatment is again through local injection of hydrocortisone, although physical measures can be successful. Addressing the (occupational) cause is important and protecting the wrist in a Futuro® wrist splint may occasionally be helpful in the short term.

Work-related upper limb disorders

This was commonly known as the repetitive strain disorder (RSD), see Box 27.3 for definition. Although acute syndromes occur in the workplace, which settle on cessation of the activity, the progression to a chronic regional pain syndrome (CRPS) is not known.

Box 27.3 Definition

A number of well-recognized musculoskeletal conditions of the work-place, which are associated with acute, cumulative and chronic 'injuries' and illnesses of soft tissue caused by mechanical stress, strain, sprain and vibration, inflammation or irritation.

Epidemiology

Facts

- Women more affected than men.
- Rare in self-employed people.
- More common in those with mundane repetitive jobs with little job satisfaction.
- Epidemic phenomena are produced in companies or even in a country by the publicity surrounding several cases in which awards were made for compensation.
- Claims can continue to rise despite improvements in the working practices.
- Numbers of soft tissue problems fell dramatically when new legislation introduced to reduce the number of dubious claims.
- Companies with Australian and European offices noted that the problem was more prevalent among Australian employees, despite the fact that all were using the same equipment.
- There was a higher incidence in seasonal workers, such as fruit pickers just before the end of the season and just before the start of their children's school holidays.
- More common among public sector employees and in those companies whose volume of work was decreasing.
- Symptoms characteristically appear through an increased working demand or a change in practice.

Diagnostic criteria

The clinical diagnosis is made by a history and findings of:

- Upper limb pain in someone whose occupation demands regular and repetitive arm activity.
- Wrist or hand—or less commonly elbow or shoulder—pain.
- Usually starts as limb discomfort accompanied by weakness.
- Leads on to localized tenderness at a tendon/nerve/enthesis in the wrist, forearm, or hand.
- Pain more commonly confined to the extensor aspect of the limb.
- Common feature is hypersensitivity of overlying structures.
- Decreased pinch grip is an important factor and 20% difference between hands is significant.
- If symptoms bilateral, a 20 Newton decrease (hand-held dynamometer) from that expected in the normal population is significant.
- Decreased fingertip sensitivity to vibration differentiates between those with genuine pain from those with functional symptoms. A 256Hz middle C tuning fork on index and middle fingers gave only 18% false positives and negatives.

The typical patient is a young or middle aged woman with a long history of arthralgia or myalgia, prolonged morning stiffness, chronic sleep disturbance, and easy fatigue and poor exercise tolerance. She may have other unrelated tender points and acrocyanosis and there is often subjective swelling of the hands along with non-dermatomal paraesthesiae (pins and needles in a limb, over and above a nerve root territory). On examination a degree of dermatographia and considerable impairment of function are present. Pain is often present on moving the neck, but the range of movement is invariably normal. Despite pain-induced muscle power testing, neurological examination is essentially normal. There is a higher prevalence of smoking among sufferers than in the normal female population, but epidemiological studies have not matched subjects for age and social class, which may thus nullify this difference.

Differential diagnosis

- Carpal tunnel syndrome.
- de Quervain's tenosynovitis.
- Lateral or medial humeral epicondylitis.
- Anterior and posterior tibial interosseous syndromes.
- Rotator cuff problems at the shoulder.

Investigations

The diagnosis is clinical and investigations should be kept to a minimum in CRPS type 1.

Amputation

Introduction

Epidemiology

Peripheral vascular disease, the major cause of amputation in the UK, is due to:
- Arteriosclerosis:
  - Hypertension.
  - Obesity.
  - Diabetes itself.
  - Hyperlipidaemia.
  - Smoking.
- Diabetes mellitus—end-stage obliterative arterial , micro-angiopathic, and neurological disease

5000 patients are referred annually in the UK for prosthetic treatment (10 000 amputations)—see Table 28.1. Upper limb amputation accounts for about 10%. Amputations from trauma and congenital limb deficiency are now uncommon, but young users will need an artificial limb for longer and may have more demanding expectations to allow them to return to an active life. Regular limb changes will be required as often as every few months during growth spurts in children.

Planning an amputation

The amputee care team should begin the rehabilitation process as soon as amputation is considered and acts through patient education, defining expectations and artificial limb fitting, as well as advising the surgeon on the choice of surgical operation and the suitability of patients for using artificial limbs. The team also helps and supports patients in the long term.

Information is the key to success, particularly on what it is like to be an amputee, of phantom limb pain and sensation and stump care. Phantom limb pain is associated with pre-operative pain, and can be reduced by sustained pain relief for at least 72 hours before surgery and 48 hours afterwards.

Amputation care

- Fitness training—to allow optimal walking, transfers and standing for long periods.
- Care of surviving limb—vital, therefore avoid hopping and jumping.
- Amputation level—critical for the expected level of independence, e.g. transtibial and transfemoral, transradial and transhumeral, knee disarticulation.
- Preservation of knee function—key to independence, eases transfers and walking energy, cosmesis.
- Increased energy costs—above and below knee amputees (vascular disease) by 120% and 55% respectively. Bilateral above knee amputees 280%.
- Prediction of walking—fitness, indication for surgery, age, stump health and length, energy costs, complications.

Table 28.1 UK amputations by age and cause

Aetiology	Age (years)					
	0–9	10–19	29–39	40–59	60–79	80+
Trauma	1	33	158	93	41	7
Vascular	2	0	17	294	1563	323
Diabetic	2	0	5	140	507	68
Infection	1	0	13	13	28	2
Malignancy	0	11	26	26	37	10

The limb fitting process

A temporary limb can be fitted within 10—14 days after surgery. The post-amputation mobility aid (PPAM) can be fitted as early as 3–4 weeks and allows compression of the stump through its air cells (thereby reducing oedema and in promoting healing) and early standing, which is useful in the elderly.

Prosthetic treatment

- Stump casting and measurement and limb prescription from the 21st post-operative day.
- Modular systems are used from the very first prescription and temporary cosmetic covers shorten delivery times.
- Gait re-education with the first prosthesis follows a common sequence (Box 28.1).

> **Box 28.1 Rehabilitation therapy sequence**
>
> - Full weight-bearing and weight transfer.
> - Walking within parallel bars, turning by stepping.
> - Walking with sticks between two parallel bars.
> - Walking with one stick between parallel bars.
> - Walking with aids out of the bars.
> - Optimal gait with minimal walking aids.

The prescription of a prosthesis has to account for the following common features, which interface with the residual limb.
- Socket structure—skeletal structure.
- Articular structures—terminal structures.
- A cosmetic covering—a suspension.

Modern prostheses incorporate design features to improve the gait cycle. The use of intelligent knees and ankle shock absorption allow a smoother gait, reduce energy costs, and resist the forces transmitted during stance and gait without serious risk of mechanical failure. Functional limb prostheses may be body powered and electronically powered features are now becoming more commonly available. A variety of silicones are used in suction and adhesion devices at the interface, but stump sheaths, called stump socks, are the commonest interface, as they provide considerable relief from shear forces.

A prosthesis has to allow sufficient height for the foot to swing through during the swing phase of the gait cycle. Therefore, heel strike at the start of the next stance phase has to be controlled very quickly, if the artificial leg is to cope with walking forces and the patient has to have the ability to achieve the correct posture and position.

Special needs

Young people with limb deficiency—particularly those with an interest in sport—require robust tensile artificial limbs with adjustable qualities and strong components, e.g. hydraulic swing-phase controls and energy storing and reducing shin/ankle/foot systems. Protective sleeves are therefore used over the prosthesis for protection, as both exo- and endoskeletal prostheses are not usually waterproof and can prove somewhat hazardous, if they get wet.

Outcomes

As in many aspects of disability, it is difficult to find a useful, easily applicable measure of progress during rehabilitation. The Harold Wood/Stanmore Scale[1] and the Guy Scales measure mobility and are currently used in the U.K. A Grise Scale is validated as a general outcome measure for amputees, but unfortunately is insensitive to change and it is this very element on which one wishes to gain most information.

Therefore, standard rehabilitation outcome measures are relevant to interventions for amputees and measures of mobility, impairment, activity and participation/quality of life used.

References

1. Hanspal RS (1991) Mobility grades in amputee rehabilitation. *Clinical Rehabilitation* **5**: 344–347.

Further reading

1. Amputee rehabilitation recommended standards and guidelines (2003). BSRM working party report, British society of rehabilitation medicine, London.
2. British Society of Rehabilitation Medicine (1999). Measuring outcome in rehabilitation medicine, BSRM Basket of measures BSRM working party report, London. In the effectness of rehabilitation: acutical review of the evidence. *Clinical rehabilitation* **13** suppl 1.
3. Turner-Stokes L and Turner-Stokes T (1997) The use of standardized outcome measures in rehabilitation centres in the UK. *Clinical Rehabilitation* **11**: 306–13.

Ageing and disability

Background

Two aspects of ageing need to be considered in physically disabled people.
- The impact of the ageing process on disabled people.
- The impact of the disability on the ageing process.

Effect of age on disability

Because of the population's increasing longevity, there is greater pressure on NHS facilities and on the need for care and intermittent rehabilitation.

Effect of disability on ageing

Are there any differences between the ageing process in disabled and able-bodied individuals? The answer is probably no, but there are specific features which seem to occur more readily in disabled people (☐ see Fig. 29.1). The most common aspect of the ageing process in physically disabled people is the appearance of degenerative joint disease, particularly in an increased prevalence of shoulder, hip, and knee osteoarthritis. Radiological changes occur in 54% of men and 58% of women. Joint pain and soreness has also been reported and decreased strength and energy levels are noted, particularly in tetraplegics.

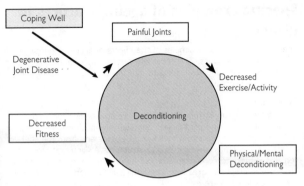

Fig. 29.1 Deconditioning

Specific examples of ageing features in disability

There are a few classic examples of the effects of ageing in people with long-standing disabilities. The most obvious example is the increasing numbers of co-morbidities leading to difficulties in concentrating on the rehabilitation process.

Spinal injuries

The effects of ageing in spinal cord injury are now being seen, as patients survive with tetra- and para-plegias. Shoulder and neck problems appear to be evident from years of wheelchair propulsion and from the effect of using the upper limbs as weight-bearing structures. A significant proportion requires surgery to correct rotator cuff lesions and there is an increased incidence in pressure sores with increasing age. Cardiopulmonary impairments develop and are evident with impaired circulation in the legs and hypertension in tetraplegics. Paraplegics have a profile consistent with the general population. Mortality increases exponentially with age, but there is an extra mortality due to spinal cord injury. However, the mortality ratio decreases with age. Whereas a 20-year-old with a spinal cord injury has a mortality 8 times higher than the general population, survivors aged 70 years have a mortality rate of only 1.5 times higher. It was reported that the causes of death mirrored the general population and that there was an association with renal failure, particularly again in tetraplegics. However, over the years, since these studies have become more widely known, renal problems have been better addressed and the mortality is much more akin to the non-disabled population.

Traumatic brain injury

There are two age-related peaks in the incidence of traumatic brain injury. In the young, injuries occur from car accidents, etc., but in the elderly they are often due to falls within the home. With multi-system failure, mobility and stability decrease and elderly people fall over more readily. This results in a higher incidence in head injuries and is a reflection more of their social and health status rather than the epidemic seen in younger people. However, as with the young, physical and cognitive changes occur to an already failing brain and there is a significant morbidity and mortality attached to traumatic brain injury in the elderly. Additionally less force is required to damage the skull bones, but elderly people somewhat paradoxically appear to recover better than expected both cognitively and physically after traumatic brain injury.

Cerebral palsy

Ambulation in people with cerebral palsy deteriorates as they approach their 5th decade. Several reasons have been postulated, but none predominates. The result, however, is that they tend to become wheelchair users even though there is no significant change in the level of spasticity or muscle power. They also are likely to complain of muscle tears and cramp-like pain, in later life. Again, the reason for this is unclear.

Post-polio syndrome

This syndrome is classically seen 20 years or so after the development of poliomyelitis-related disability. People with poliomyelitis learn to cope with their disability while young, but after a while, they notice increasing difficulty carrying out tasks which were previously straightforward and further investigation shows denervation in the muscles supplied by the affected anterior horn cells. In simplistic terms, it would appear that their lower motor neurones 'burn out' after years of 'overwork' and this possibly represents the effect of normal ageing on a depleted population of anterior horn cells, which have had to supply an expanded number of motor units. There is no evidence that this syndrome has been caused by an awakening of any viral activity in the disease.

Mobility

The normal ageing process changes one's gait throughout life. As one passes from an infant's gait—which is wide-based and involves pelvic rotation—myelination allows better neuromuscular transmission and growth of bones allows an adult-type gait at around the age of the 5th birthday. Serially, as one gets older, balance mechanisms become less efficient and one naturally shortens the stride length in walking and increases the proportion of the stance phase during the gait cycle during the 7th decade of life. This ensures better stability while walking, but results in decreased walking speed and shortened strides. Increased loading of joints leads to degenerative change in the hip and knee. Similarly, the vectors of the forces coming up the lower limb during this altered gait cycle lead to mild flexion of the trunk, which over years gives the stooped posture of elderly people. This puts increasing pressure on the articulating facet joints in the lumbar spine, and hence the stiffness and discomfort that can develop.

Conclusion

There is an increased incidence in musculo-skeletal disease, in strokes, in neurodegenerative disease, and in cancers with increasing age. As already stated, the rehabilitation of older people is complicated by the presence of co-morbidities, which slow the rehabilitation process down and is one of the major differences between rehabilitating the elderly population from a younger disabled population. The needs of both populations are similar in severe disability, as is the impact of the disability. However, there are distinct differences between the support available, the expectations of the individuals compared to the younger population, and very often the aims of rehabilitation. The OPCS survey in 1988[1] showed that 32% of people with disabilities living in private households were aged 75 years and over; 26% were between the ages of 75 and 64; and 19% between the ages of 55 and 64.

References

1. Martin J, Meltzer H, and Elliot D (1988). *OPCS Report 1, The Prevalence of Disability Among Adults.* HMSO, London.

Further reading

1. Andrews K (1987). *Rehabilitation of the older adult.* Edward Arnold, London.
2. Calne DB, Comi G, Crippa D et al. (1989). *Parkinsonism and ageing.* Raven Press, New York.

Index

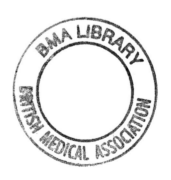